THE
HIDDEN
FACE OF
SHYNESS

THE HIDDEN FACE OF SHYNESS

UNDERSTANDING & OVERCOMING SOCIAL ANXIETY

FRANKLIN SCHNEIER, M.D., AND
LAWRENCE WELKOWITZ, PH.D.

AVON BOOKS ◆ NEW YORK

Permissions are listed on page v, which constitutes an extension of the copyright page

THE HIDDEN FACE OF SHYNESS is an original publication of Avon Books. This work has never before appeared in book form.

AVON BOOKS, INC.
1350 Avenue of the Americas
New York, New York 10019

Copyright © 1996 by Franklin R Schneier, M D. and Lawrence A Welkowitz, Ph D.
Published by arrangement with the authors
Library of Congress Catalog Card Number: 96-33699
ISBN: 0-380-78399-1
www.avonbooks.com

Library of Congress Cataloging in Publication Data:

Schneier, Franklin.
     The hidden face of shyness : understanding and overcoming social anxiety / Franklin Schneier and Lawrence Welkowitz.
         p. cm.
Includes bibliographical references and index.
1 Anxiety. 2. Bashfulness I. Welkowitz, Lawrence II Title.
BF575 A6S34   1996   96-33699
155 2'32—dc20   CIP

First Avon Books Trade Paperback Printing: September 1996

AVON TRADEMARK REG U S PAT OFF AND IN OTHER COUNTRIES, MARCA REGISTRADA, HECHO EN U S A

Printed in the U S.A.

OPM 10 9 8 7 6 5 4

To Carol, Mary Ann, and Annika

ACKNOWLEDGMENTS

We wish to express our appreciation to Michael Liebowitz. In addition to reviewing a portion of a draft of this book, he has been a mentor and key collaborator in our study of social phobia, an area of research he helped put on the map. We also are indebted to the following colleagues who have generously read and provided critical review of parts of drafts of this book, and who have helped us to develop many of our ideas about social anxiety over the years: Donald Klein, Jack Gorman, Abby Fyer, Sharon Davies, Mary Guardino, Susan Clarvit, and Randall Marshall. Additionally, our research on this topic would not have been possible without the help of the dedicated staffs of the Anxiety Disorders Clinic and the Biological Studies Unit at New York State Psychiatric Institute.

Special thanks to our agent, Sheree Bykofsky, and our editor, Stephen S. Power, for their wise guidance throughout this project.

We are extremely grateful for the valuable comments of our friends and family members who read parts of earlier drafts: Manuel Vargas; Jim Rousmaniere; Roger and Ann Sweet; Kathleen Bollerud; Gertrude and H. Oliver Schneier; and Carol Rosenthal, whose editorial and emotional support far exceeded what F.S. or any other spouse could deserve.

Finally, we owe a tremendous amount to our patients, whose stories of courage and personal growth have inspired us to write this book.

CONTENTS

THE
HIDDEN
FACE OF
SHYNESS

I

INTRODUCTION

1

WHAT IS SOCIAL PHOBIA?

Something strange happened to Harry. His heart started racing out of control, his face felt flushed, and his hands shook so that he nearly spilled his drink. All of a sudden, he couldn't remember what he had been about to say, and when he did remember, he found it difficult to get out the words. Everything around him seemed unreal.

You might suppose Harry feared he was experiencing a heart attack or a stroke, but neither illness concerned him. Instead, he worried that the people around him would think he was awkward and pathetic; instead of wanting to call for help, he just wanted to disappear. This odd scenario makes perfect sense given one additional bit of information: Harry was about to offer a toast at his friend's wedding. He was experiencing intense stage fright.

In surveys of people's greatest fears, fear of public speaking often ranks number one, even greater than fear of dying. Most of us are familiar with at least mild fear of embarrassment yet the damage social fears can do to people's lives remains little-known, the hidden face of shyness. Those who suffer extreme shyness only occasionally, such as when giving a toast at a wedding, may experience only a few moments of terror. For many others, social fears creep into more common situations, such as approaching someone at a party, or speaking up in a meeting. And for millions of Americans, the same paralyzing fear of embarrassment erupts every day—sitting down to lunch, approaching a boss, or even talking with a friend.

In our clinical practices, we often see the severe side of this hidden face of shyness, the terrific pain and missed opportunities of its victims. We will tell the stories of a veteran actor whose career is ruined by stage fright; a child so shy he will not speak at all; a macho detective racked by anxiety for weeks whenever he has to testify in court; an attractive woman who rejects dinner dates because she fears her hand will tremble if she is seen eating. When social anxiety causes persistent distress or interferes with life's activities, it is considered a disorder known as "social phobia."

Many otherwise well adjusted people, who consider themselves to be only mildly or not at all shy, may be handicapped in more subtle ways by the anxiety they experience in certain social or public situations. They may have hesitated long enough to miss out on chances to make a new friend or business contact. Social anxiety may have influenced them to avoid giving a talk or even to forgo a career that would require public speaking. Now both mild and severe forms of social anxiety can be helped.

The terms "shyness" and "social anxiety" mean different things to different people; we will use them interchangeably in this book to refer to a variety of social and performance fears. The term "social phobia," however, is more strictly defined. In social phobia, fear of embarrassment or humiliation is excessive and persistent, and it causes a sufferer to feel great distress or to avoid social or public situations. The fears in social phobia may be limited to one important situation, such as running meetings at work, or may even interfere with everyday activities, such as going to the market or making a phone call.

Mental health professionals have only recently recognized that social phobia is very common, causes a surprising amount of suffering, and is sometimes incapacitating. This new awareness has led to an explosion of research into the causes and treatment of both milder social anxiety and social phobia. Social phobia, it turns out, is a complicated beast. We will discuss its links to our evolutionary history, our body and brain chemistries, our life experiences, our daily social habits, the characteristic ways in which we think about ourselves and others, and the values of our society at large.

In the history of medical science, study of a disorder has often led to new understandings of normal functioning. For example, the discovery of insulin treatment for diabetes led to the recognition that diabetes is a disorder of a normal system in which blood sugar is regulated by insulin, a hormone released by the pancreas. So it is not surprising that recent discoveries in social phobia have important implications for understanding and coping with milder forms of social anxiety as well. Social phobia seems to be a result of the normal human social anxiety system run amok.

*   *   *

We became interested in these problems as we were completing our professional training in the mid-1980s in psychiatry (F.S.) and psychology (L.W.). The term "social phobia" had been added to the official diagnostic manual of the American Psychiatric Association only in 1979, and in 1985 the publication of a scholarly article titled "Social Phobia: A Review of a Neglected Anxiety Disorder" by psychiatrist Michael Liebowitz called attention to the need for research on this problem. It was as if a spotlight had been switched on, for we had been aware that some of our patients suffered from serious shyness or embarrassment, but we knew of no specific treatment approaches for this problem—in fact, they barely existed at the time. We each joined Liebowitz's research group at the Anxiety Disorders Clinic of New York State Psychiatric Institute, and we have been studying social phobia and its treatment ever since.

In our research and our clinical practices, we have seen hundreds of people suffering from excessive fears of embarrassment. The fear is puzzling to our patients because they recognize that its intensity is out of proportion to the realities of their situations. Some sufferers are troubled most by particular social anxiety symptoms, such as blushing or excessive sweating. Others are most concerned by the consequences of their fear and avoidance, such as depression or loneliness, problems on the job, or difficulties forming relationships. What these people share, however, is our universal concern about what others will think of us—taken to the extreme.

Although social phobia sufferers experience the same kinds of symptoms anyone might feel as a result of "normal" embarrassment or self-consciousness, they are not the "worried well." Beyond just feeling distress, they are actually missing out on opportunities to fulfill their potential, both socially and at work.

Chloe, for example, passed up college to avoid the terror she experienced when teachers called on her to speak in the classroom. Todd had twice ended promising serious relationships with understanding women rather than face the humiliating chance that anxiety would prevent him from being able to perform sexually. Jackie managed to keep up appearances of functioning well while feeling great shame over secretly "self-medicating" her social anxiety with alcohol. Ted constructed his life around his fears, passing up job promotions that would have required him to speak in public. For others, the problems are less pervasive. Sufferers whose anxiety is limited to a specific situation, such as performing onstage, may lead full and successful lives while avoiding their feared situation—if they can get away with avoiding it. Ironically, they may even be extroverts who relish being with people outside their feared situation.

Most people with social phobia, however, try to avoid drawing attention to themselves. Even when the attention is positive, such as a serenade of "Happy Birthday," people with social phobia usually prefer to fade into the background. But becoming part of the scenery can make it difficult to meet people and keep friends, or to get recognition for work achievements.

Another result of this reticence is that the topic of social phobia is rarely broached in public. The quiet suffering of shy people has not been a "hot" topic for the news media, but the sheer number of persons so adversely affected by social phobia calls out for more public attention. A recent survey sponsored by the National Institute of Mental Health showed that social phobia has afflicted more than 13 percent of adults in the United States, making it one of the most common mental disorders.

Social phobia does not discriminate. Although it was once thought primarily to be a problem of the upper classes, it now has been shown to affect persons in all segments of society. For the famous or the powerful, public speaking anxiety, or stage fright, can derail high-profile careers. For others, social fears can frustrate ambitions (thus sparing them the trouble of ever becoming famous or powerful) and limit social activities, denying them even the most basic satisfactions in life. Social phobia is most common in adolescence and young adulthood, but it affects people of all ages. For the child with social phobia, school can be a daily terror. For the middle-aged divorcée faced with dating for the first time in decades, it can lead to isolation and depression.

While we commonly see the distress social phobia causes our patients, we have become more aware, through writing this book, of the huge numbers of people who struggle with their own milder versions of social fears. Stories suddenly start to flow whenever we mention our area of research. One of us (F.S.) was chatting at a party recently with a seemingly gregarious, risk-taking entrepreneur when the topic of this book came up. He sheepishly confessed to feeling terribly uncomfortable at parties, and F.S. told him how invisible his social anxiety had been. The next person F.S. encountered was a successful lawyer who declared that nobody could ever get *him* to give a public speech. He added with a chuckle, however, that his wife was a professor who loved speaking to huge audiences but trembled with fear at the thought of inviting a couple over for an intimate dinner. Feeling on a roll, F.S. asked his next conversation partner, a local politician, if any of his colleagues seemed to suffer from fears of embarrassment. "No," he said with a smile, "but if you heard some of the things they say, you'd agree that they really *should* be embarrassed."

Although social anxiety is widespread, affecting people in (nearly) all segments of society, surprisingly little was known about social phobia until the past decade. One reason psychiatrists and psychologists had learned little about it is that they did not see much of it in their practices—persons with social phobia rarely seek treatment. Not surprisingly for a disorder of embarrassment and humiliation, some sufferers are ashamed of their fears—or worry that their complaints will not be taken seriously by a therapist, that they'll be told they're "just a little shy." We have received sadly eloquent letters from people who could write of the great pain social phobia had caused them but were unable to risk the embarrassment of telling their stories in person, even to a therapist.

Interest in social phobia among mental health professionals has picked up dramatically in the past decade. Clinicians are now recognizing the problem in their practices, and researchers are developing and testing a variety of new treatment approaches. For us, it has been an exciting time to be studying social anxiety and a rewarding time to be treating people with problems in this area.

Unfortunately, the spread of knowledge from the research clinic to the general public can be slow. Add the stigma that still plagues mental health problems in general and the acute embarrassment of persons with social phobia in particular, and the process of getting the word out can be frustrating. Any TV talk show host would be able to find more people eager to tell millions of viewers why they like to terrorize their spouses than people willing to tell about their private struggles with serious fear of embarrassment.

In this book we recount the stories we have been privileged to learn from our patients and clients. We will try to put these stories in meaningful perspective using the wealth of findings of dedicated researchers and clinicians in the field and our own, admittedly premature speculations about what we cannot yet know for sure. We also will offer both a specific program that readers can use to overcome their social fears and facts about effective professional treatments that are available for social phobia.

THE MOST HUMAN FEAR

Prepare a face to meet the faces that you meet.

T. S. Eliot

At age twenty-five, Lydia came to our clinic because she had decided that she could no longer afford to wait to grow out of her fears of embarrassment. It had always taken her a long time to overcome her initial shyness and warm up to people. As a child, Lydia had moved frequently with her family to follow her father's job opportunities, and each time it took her as long as a year to develop some new friends and some level of comfort in her new home.

In classroom situations, Lydia used to avoid speaking up as long as her teachers would allow. She always felt her answers might not be good enough, that others might make fun of her if she made a mistake or stumbled over her words. At home, her parents were quiet and caring but very protective, and they had discouraged her from playing with other children on her street. She did manage to develop a few good friends, and she did well enough in school, but during high school things gradually changed for the worse.

Lydia increasingly felt herself automatically clamming up in groups, although she wanted to connect with people, to be spontaneous like some of her classmates. She always let others start conversations, fearing that if she initiated them the other person might be uninterested. She felt very uncomfortable at dances and parties.

When boys asked her out, she often would find excuses to say no.

Dating was not the carefree fun it appeared to be in the movies, and she wondered how others managed to find things to talk about. Lydia recounted memories of dates in which minutes went by painfully slowly, literally without a word of actual conversation, but with fearful thoughts racing through her mind. Following a difficult social situation, Lydia would play the critic. She would review her social miscues in agonizing detail, berate herself for her failures, and wonder if she would ever feel more comfortable.

Over time, Lydia did make some gradual progress on her own. In college she forced herself to socialize even when fearful, recognizing that the exposure was good for her. She pushed herself to take some chances, trying to say what was on her mind and to see how others reacted. Usually the results turned out better than she had feared, and her conversational skills had definitely improved. Still, she felt socially limited and lonely.

Now she was struggling with adapting to a new job. During informal meetings with her boss, a critical man, her social fears flared up again. What if she stumbled over her words or appeared anxious? If her face twitched from anxiety, she wondered if her boss would think she was on drugs. She would worry about an upcoming meeting for days. Even after it had gone reasonably well, Lydia tended to consider herself lucky, and she feared that the next meeting would be a disaster.

The final straw for Lydia was that her fears were becoming worse again, even spreading into new situations. She was avoiding parties more and felt she was missing out on opportunities for friendships. She knew it was ridiculous, but she even found her heart palpitating when she encountered a middle-aged neighbor as she entered her apartment building. She feared that if the neighbor tried to start a conversation he would notice her shaky voice and think she was a nervous wreck.

Lydia was experiencing social phobia's core feature, excessive and irrational fear of embarrassment or humiliation. These fearful thoughts frequently go along with physical symptoms of anxiety and actual avoidance of social situations, and combined they form the typical syndrome. No single feature of this syndrome is serious or abnormal when it occurs occasionally, but when the excessive fear and anxiety persist, causing a person to forgo important activities and resulting in significant impairment of social life or work, the result is considered a disorder.

VARIATIONS ON EMBARRASSMENT

The central fear in social phobia is not so much a fear of other people as it is a fear of embarrassment. Embarrassment is one of the more socially sophisticated human emotions. Unlike anger, pleasure, or simple fear, this emotion requires a capacity for self-consciousness that is not present in most animals or even in very young children. It requires the ability to put yourself in someone else's shoes and to take a look at yourself through another's eyes. The thought processes that accompany embarrassment typically involve awareness of how you might be evaluated negatively by others and concern about the consequences of such an evaluation.

Being in an embarrassing situation can call into play a host of healthy or unhealthy coping strategies. These range from humor or a simple apology to awkward silence ("The safest thing to do is nothing at all"), self-denigration ("I'll put myself down before they can do it"), combativeness ("The best defense is a good offense"), or flight ("They can't hurt me if they can't find me"). Over time, a person's characteristic responses can take on an automatic quality, so that they occur like reflexes.

On a biological level, embarrassment is related to more instinctive physiological and behavioral reactions, such as freezing with fear, blushing, "sheepish" grinning, and intermittently gazing downward to avoid eye contact. These familiar nonverbal responses automatically send a message. That message communicates lower social status, and it appears to have an ancient evolutionary source. As we will explain later, the behavior of human embarrassment is strikingly similar to certain "appeasement" behaviors that maintain social order in other species, such as monkeys. In a sense, for both man and animal, the behaviors signal a vital message to another individual: "I am no threat to you. I am subservient to you, so you should not harm me."

Only humans, however, build on this primal response rich layers of thought, social rules, and complex feelings. Although the experience of embarrassment, humiliation, or feeling criticized is common to all of us, individuals vary tremendously in respect to how easily embarrassment is provoked, its intensity, and its effects. These feelings also vary in the same person over a lifetime. One of the earliest forms of social anxiety is the stranger anxiety that babies normally experience between six and twenty months of age, when seeing a strange face may cause fright and crying. While babies grow out of this phase, those who exhibit a more extreme fear of strangers have been shown to be more likely to develop persistent shyness and inhibition as they grow older.

True concerns about embarrassment appear more clearly after age three, when children begin to acquire the capacity to understand the abstract idea of a "self" that exists over time. Only then can they begin to suffer the consequences of trying to see themselves as others might. These social concerns often intensify with the added social expectations of adolescence or with other stressful situations, such as moving to a new town and trying to make a new set of friends. Social fears can also be activated in adulthood when disturbing life events, such as divorce—or even a positive event such as a job promotion—force a person into the demanding new social situations of dating or public speaking.

Many people with social anxiety find their fears triggered by particular social and public situations. Some commonly feared situations are performing onstage; dealing with a boss or other authority figure; being in a place that requires making small talk, such as a party; or simply being observed in a public place, such as while eating in a restaurant or just waiting on line for a bus. In all of these situations the underlying fear revolves around embarrassment or some kind of negative evaluation by others: "She will think less of me," "They will say I'm not good enough," "He will think I'm stupid and not hire me."

Cognitive therapists have noted the gap between these individuals' beliefs (that they are socially incompetent or on the brink of social catastrophe) and their actual social skills (which are often excellent). In other words, some people who are quite able to perform in front of others or make charming conversation at a party nevertheless see themselves as unable to say or do the right thing. The same individuals recognize, however, that this negative view is exaggerated or irrational. For some other persons with social phobia, social skills actually do seem to disappear when they get anxious.

Some people don't worry about saying or doing the wrong thing; they are just uncomfortable when others look at them. They may worry that people will notice signs of their discomfort. Physical symptoms like blushing, a racing heart, and perspiration sometimes become the main focus of the problem—as was the case with Anne, whose frequent and unpredictable blushing led her to avoid visiting people out of fear they would think her strange; and Vance, who feared his job as a construction foreman would "dissolve" in the sweat that dripped from his brow during meetings. How do you concentrate on what others are saying when your attention is riveted on monitoring not only your own physical symptoms but others' reactions to them as well? These people are trying to watch all the acts in a three-ring circus. The distraction of the physical symptoms leads to worse social performance, which increases fear and anxiety symptoms, which distracts from concentration and performance, and so on in a spiraling vicious cycle.

THE PRICE OF FEAR

Socially anxious people often develop elaborate strategies for either escaping or avoiding feared situations. Carla developed increasingly creative excuses to avoid the lunchroom at work, dating situations, and any social gathering where food would be served, all to avoid revealing that her hands trembled when she ate in front of others. Roger was a middle-level business manager with an intense fear of public speaking. In order to create an excuse for turning down invitations to lead training workshops, he arranged extra paperwork for himself. He avoided running these workshops at the cost of not being promoted to positions of greater prestige and income. In sum, many socially anxious people pay a high price for the short-term relief they get by avoiding their feared situations.

This avoidance also has serious long-term consequences. A study that followed up shy and nonshy children, thirty years after they were first categorized, found that men who had been shy tended to marry several years later than nonshy men. They also entered careers several years later and achieved less. Women who had been shy were less likely to work outside the home. In another study, among people attending a clinic for treatment of social phobia, 69 percent believed that their anxiety interfered with social relationships, 85 percent reported interference with school, and 92 percent reported interference with work. Adults with social phobia have consistently been shown to have lower rates of marriage than would otherwise be expected.

With such impairment affecting such large numbers of people, social phobia adds up to a considerably bigger problem than was once thought. In addition to the recent National Institute of Mental Health survey estimating that more than 30 million adults in the U.S. have experienced the pain of social phobia, other studies have reported high rates of particular "types" of social phobia. Psychiatrist Murray Stein found that 31 percent of people surveyed in a Canadian city considered themselves to be much more nervous than other people with respect to public speaking.

These impressive statistics still do not portray the full scope of the problem. As a friend and colleague has said, "We all have social phobia." He was exaggerating, of course, although when even Madonna has complained of social anxiety, who can deny at least a brush with it? For some, social anxiety is only an uncomfortable experience of butterflies in the stomach before going to a party or speaking in public, while for others it may be severe and persistent anxiety that leads to intolerable suffering and loneliness. Because social anxiety seems to occur on a continuum of severity, we can use the lessons we have learned about treating severe forms of social phobia to help people cope with everyday social anxiety as well.

SOCIAL PHOBIA ACROSS PLACE AND TIME

Social phobia also appears to be common outside North America, and careful surveys have been done on at least five continents. In some places, intriguing cultural variants of the problem appear to exist. In Japan and Korea, a condition called *taijin kyofusho* was first described in the 1920s, independently of Western psychiatry. Although this disorder seems to overlap with the Western concept of social phobia, persons with *taijin kyofusho* often fear that they will make *others* become uncomfortable and embarrassed—by looking at people too directly or by emitting offensive body odors, for example. This concern with embarrassing others is less common in Western societies. Cultural attitudes seem to shape powerfully the form and severity of social anxiety.

Social phobia is hardly unique to our era. The ancient Greek physician Hippocrates described a patient who "through bashfulness, suspicion and timorousness will not be seen abroad. . . . He dare not come in company, for fear he should be misused, disgraced, overshoot himself in gestures or speeches, or be sick; he thinks every man observes him . . ." Many ages and cultures have acknowledged social anxiety as a problematic condition, but it was never defined as a specific disorder until the early twentieth century. At that time the French psychiatrist Pierre Janet used the term *"phobie des situations sociales"* to describe patients who feared being observed by others in such situations as speaking, playing the piano, or writing. Sigmund Freud had surprisingly little to say about social anxiety, however, and with the rise of psychoanalytic theory in the twentieth century, social phobia receded into a more general category of phobias. These avoidance behaviors were theorized to be "defensive" reactions against one's own disturbing aggressive or sexual urges.

Only in recent years has social phobia been widely accepted as a specific disorder, distinct in its origins and characteristics, and responding to particular treatments. In the 1960s, British psychiatrist Isaac Marks called attention to social phobia as a condition in which people fear a variety of situations in which other people may look at them or form an opinion of them. Marks recognized the social and work difficulties that these individuals experienced as a result of avoiding feared activities.

Marks also discovered that social phobia stood apart from other kinds of phobias in respect to the age at which it typically became a problem. Unlike specific phobias, such as fear of spiders or fear of the dark, which typically begin in early childhood, or agoraphobia (fear of places where escape could be difficult in event of an unexpected panic attack), which typically begins in one's twenties, the average age of onset for social phobia is the mid-teens. (Although shyness may be present from early childhood, truly impairing social phobia is more likely to develop in adolescence.) This was the first evidence that social phobia might be very different from other phobias, with unique features that might respond to specialized treatments. More recent work has further defined the demographic, psychological, physical, and genetic characteristics that distinguish social anxiety and social phobia from other forms of anxiety.

American psychiatry built on Marks's definition of social phobia and established criteria for the diagnosis. The official psychiatric diagnostic manual, DSM-IV, defines social phobia as: "A persistent fear of one or more situations . . . in which the person is exposed to possible scrutiny by others and fears that he or she may do something or act in a way that will be humiliating or embarrassing." The current definition includes persons with "generalized" fears across numerous social and performance situations, as well as persons with discrete fears limited to one or a few situations. It restricts the diagnosis to persons for whom social fear and avoidance result in impairment in social or work functioning, or cause extreme distress.

SOME FACES OF SHYNESS

Some typical activities feared in social phobia, which we will discuss in more detail later, include:

Public speaking. This is the most common of all social fears, and it often interferes with work, full participation in church or civic groups, or even being able to offer a toast at a family celebration. The phobia may occur even if the person has mastered the materials to be presented, learned public speaking techniques, and successfully given talks in the past.

Performance onstage (or stage fright). Musicians, actors, and other performers often become anxious before or during a performance, fearing they will make a mistake or that their anxiety will be evident to others. Typically, "butterflies" clear up after the performance starts. When the anxiety is intense or leads to avoidance, however, it can be debilitating. Superior skills, public acclaim, and long experience may build confidence, but they didn't provide immunity from social phobia for such performers as Barbra Streisand or Sir Laurence Olivier, who made public their career-limiting struggles with stage fright.

Dealing with authority figures. Here the feared audience is concentrated into a single powerful person. This problem commonly occurs in dealings with a boss, a teacher, or even a clerk in a store. The person with social phobia may worry excessively about making a minor request; he or she may assume that making the request will be extremely awkward, that rejection is likely to occur, and that any failure will be humiliating.

Eating and drinking. Most people don't consider eating or drinking with others to be a performance event, unless they happen to be the chef. For some people, however, the act of taking a bite of food or sipping a drink in front of another person takes on the quality of a solo act in a sold-out stadium. The main fear is often of spilling a drink or of trembling so much that others will notice they are anxious or think they are crazy. For some, this fear extends to all public eating, while for others it may happen only when they are with people they wish to impress.

Writing (or scriptophobia). Like people who fear eating or drinking in public, people who fear writing in public usually believe that their hands will shake and that others will notice and think badly of them. In most instances the sufferer is able to work around this fear by signing checks or other paperwork in private, but in some professional activities this phobia can be disabling.

Dating. As unusual as fear of eating or writing in public may seem, having some anxiety about dating would appear perfectly reasonable to most of us. But whereas most people have experienced some fear or hesitation around dating, the fear tends to be transient and doesn't seriously prevent them from seeking romantic relationships. Persistent and extreme dating fear and avoidance are somewhat more common among men, who are more likely to feel that it is their responsibility to request a date. Some of these individuals will rarely date unless they can be assured of not being rejected, and their lack of social activity often leads to depression and further isolation.

Public bathrooms. Using a public bathroom is generally considered neither a public performance nor a social event, but for some it can bring on the same kind of fear response. This fear is also most common among men, and typically involves self-consciousness about using a urinal in the presence of others. The resulting anxiety response includes an involuntary tightening of muscles that control bladder function, making it more difficult to urinate. These men worry that others will notice that they are not urinating and will wonder why. To avoid "scrutiny," men with this fear may avoid public rest rooms and suffer painfully full bladders at work, sneak into rest rooms they know to be unoccupied, or use toilet stalls rather than urinals.

Sexual performance. The bedroom is transformed into a theater, and the bed a stage, for persons with this problem. The fear is that attempts to become sexually aroused or to reach orgasm will fail, and this will result in humiliation. The resulting anxiety does not improve functioning, of course, as the fearful mind again seems at war with an uncooperative body.

Taking a test. If a person with social phobia can turn the most pleasurable activities into an examination, then what of a test itself? It depends. Persons whose fears center on how they physically appear to others often have no problem taking a written test, and may actually depend on tests to demonstrate abilities they have difficulty displaying in the classroom or in an interview. For others, however, tests are a phobic performance situation. They may anticipate exams with hours of intense worry, and during exams they may experience physical symptoms of nausea or palpitations and thoughts of failure, which distract them and worsen performance.

Revealing symptoms of anxiety. This category includes fears of sweating, blushing, trembling, voice problems, or vomiting in public. The common fear is that others will notice the symptom and think badly of the sufferer. In fact, the feared symptom is usually either unlikely to occur, unlikely to be noticed, or unlikely to cause an objective observer to think badly of anyone. Fear of developing the physical anxiety symptom causes heightened awareness of other minor body sensations and creates more fear, beginning a vicious cycle.

Social encounters in general. Many individuals experience fear and anxiety generalized to most social and public situations. These people frequently believe that their social performance will fall below others' expectations. As a result, they experience discomfort when going to parties, attending meetings, talking with strangers or acquaintances, leaving messages on answering machines, or even just being seen in public. People with generalized social anxiety sometimes even build their lives around avoiding contact with unfamiliar people by working the night shift or shopping at odd hours, when there are fewer people around. Among all the types of social phobia, persons with the generalized type tend to suffer the most impairment.

Social phobia may also take the following forms:

Selective mutism. Social phobia sometimes first becomes apparent in the form of this relatively rare disorder, in which young children do not speak at all in school, even to classmates. It may be transient or it can persist for years. Teachers and peers may initially believe that the child is mentally retarded or vocally disabled, but testing reveals normal verbal skills and intelligence, and parents report that the child speaks normally at home. It has recently been shown that most of these children suffer from social phobia, fearing, for example, that their voices will sound funny to others. The recognition that social phobia often underlies this problem has opened up new possibilities for treatment.

Social phobia due to a medical condition. Certain medical conditions, embarrassing because they are noticeable to others, may bring on anxiety and avoidance in people who never had problems with social anxiety before. For example, some (but not all) persons with a tremor due to Parkinson's disease or with severe acne may try to avoid being seen in public, fearing humiliation. When social anxiety is focused exclusively on such an embarrassing medical condition, the diagnosis of social phobia technically does not apply. Such a person might benefit, however, from the same treatments used for social phobia.

TELLING SOCIAL PHOBIA APART FROM OTHER PROBLEMS

It is not really possible to discuss social phobia without considering some of the other problems with which it keeps company. People with social phobia have higher rates of other emotional disorders than would be expected by chance. Given that social phobia tends to begin at an early age, it seems to increase the risk of developing such problems as alcohol abuse, depression, or eating disorders.

Social phobia sometimes may be difficult to tell apart from other problems that cause people to fear or avoid social situations. Alcoholism often leads to eventual social withdrawal. Alternatively, some persons with underlying social phobia begin to overuse alcohol or another drug after discovering that (initially, at least) it seems to dissolve their social anxiety. Sometimes what starts out as occasional "self-medication" with alcohol becomes an uncontrollable habit that ultimately wreaks greater havoc than the original social anxiety. Abuse of other drugs, such as marijuana, can also bring on extreme self-consciousness in susceptible individuals.

The overlap between depression and social phobia also can be considerable. Many people with social phobia, after years of relentless struggles against unwanted social fears, become seriously depressed. In persons without undue social anxiety, however, major depression alone may lead to a lack of social interest and pleasure, which may result in their avoiding social events. Unlike persons with true social phobia who yearn to be more comfortable around people, these persons are not anxious around others; they have simply lost all interest in being with people.

Superficially, social phobia might seem similar to **paranoia,** in which a person may also avoid social contacts and be very concerned about what others are thinking and saying about him or her. There are two major differences here, however. First, the paranoid person doesn't fear embarrassment, but instead typically believes that he or she is being singled out by others with harmful intent. Second, the paranoid person maintains a *fixed belief* that others think badly of him, while the socially anxious person recognizes that his or her excessive fear of embarrassment is the main problem.

Panic attacks, sudden surges of extreme anxiety, may occur in social phobia, but **panic disorder** is a different condition. In social phobia, any panic attacks that occur are related in some way to fears of embarrassment. In panic disorder, attacks are usually unrelated to social fears, and they may appear out of the blue. People with panic disorder often fear they could die or pass out due to a panic attack, and they are usually comforted by having familiar people around. People with social phobia, in contrast, usually recognize that their anxiety is not physically dangerous, and they invariably prefer to be alone or to be anonymous in a crowd during an attack.

Not surprisingly, social phobia often occurs together with other conditions in which people are excessively concerned about their appearance. People with eating disorders such as anorexia nervosa, even if they are objectively below average weight, often fear that others will think badly of them because they are too fat. People with body dysmorphic disorder are preoccupied with a small or unnoticeable defect in their appearance, so that a tiny bump on the nose may seem like a horribly embarrassing deformity.

Finally, there has been some philosophical debate over whether it makes more sense to think of social phobia as a *state,* which may come and go over a lifetime, or as a more constant personality *trait.* In real life, such states and traits inevitably overlap. When social avoidance traits are extreme, they are known as "avoidant personality disorder." Persons with social phobia often feel that their avoidance symptoms are a deeply ingrained part of their personality, but recent research has shown that even what seem to be personality features can be surprisingly changeable with treatment.

Individuals with avoidant personality, like those with social phobia, are disturbed by their lack of relationships, but they may fail to recognize that the cause of this difficulty is their own behavior. They may even feel justified in avoiding social activities, thinking "Why would anybody want to socialize when others can be so critical and unreliable?" Individuals with social phobia instead blame themselves for their troubles. They are distressed over having fears and anxieties that keep them away from potentially pleasurable and rewarding activities. They want to get out, to move on, to feel better.

II

The Faces
of Social
Anxiety

3

FEAR OF PUBLIC SPEAKING

"Oh, Lord, I [Moses] am not a man of words ... for I am slow of speech and of a slow tongue...." And the Lord said ... *"I will be with thy mouth, and teach thee what thou shalt speak."*

Exodus 4:10–12

The human brain is a wonderful thing. It operates from the moment you're born, until the first time you get up to make a speech.

Howard Goshorn

BARBARA

Barbara, a 45-year-old banker, wife, and mother, came to our clinic seeking relief from the horrendous feelings she got whenever she had to lead meetings. Her hands would get clammy, her face would blush and twitch, and her heart would pound. The same feelings happened when she ate with a group of people, so she had picked up the habit of eating lunch alone at her desk. Meeting strangers was sometimes also difficult, but once she broke the ice, Barbara was able to build wonderful and close friendships. She considered herself to be strong and reliable outside of group situations. In our first session, Barbara's anxiety symptoms were not apparent at all, and she explained that her fears didn't surface much at all in one-on-one situations, especially when she felt the other person was understanding.

23

Unlike many of the patients we see, Barbara seemed at first to have an obvious underlying cause for her fears. As a young child she had been teased maliciously about her severe stuttering, and she had often felt humiliated. Barbara grew out of the stuttering completely, and she gradually lost all self-consciousness about her speech. When Barbara's fears of humiliation flared up in her early twenties, however, they were not triggered by renewed concern about the stuttering. Instead, she feared that people would notice her blushing and twitching when she had to speak in front of a group, and she worried that they would think she was incompetent.

Barbara volunteered to participate in a social phobia research study testing the effectiveness of treatment with the medication Nardil (we will discuss medication treatments for social phobia in more detail in chapter 19). Over the sixteen-week course of the study she showed clear improvement, becoming completely free of anxiety symptoms while speaking in public and socializing. Her new command of meetings at work was noticeable enough for a couple of friends to begin calling her "The New and Improved" Barbara.

She still found herself worrying a bit before upcoming meetings that anxiety might interfere, however. We decided to continue the medication beyond the first sixteen weeks to see if she might completely "unlearn" some of her fears over a longer period of treatment. We hoped this would give her the best chance to maintain improvement after we discontinued the medication. After about six months of treatment, in which she gained more confidence, we decreased and then discontinued the medicine without any loss of her new ability to speak in public and socialize, and we parted ways.

We often wonder how our patients fare after leaving treatment. Occasionally former patients will call just to say hello and to let us know that they have continued to do well. More often someone will call during a period of recurrent problems to look into the possibility of getting some additional treatment. Most often, though, people who improve during treatment go off into their lives, and we don't hear from them again. We rarely learn if their personal progress has continued or stalled. So a year after Barbara left treatment, it was very satisfying to hear from one of our research assistants that he had seen her . . . on television as a contestant on *Jeopardy!*

THE TOUGH GUY

One of the most common misconceptions about social anxiety is that it always goes along with being generally timid and insecure, that behind every trembling hand is an incompetent, fear-ridden bundle of nerves. Ted did not fit that image. At forty, this police detective was trim, muscular, handsome, and authoritative. As we discussed his situation, he was the picture of self-assurance. He was cool, calm, and collected in his speech. His work was dangerous and sometimes violent, but he could live with those risks. What he could no longer tolerate was his fear of public speaking.

Ted would go to great lengths to avoid testifying in court if he expected more than ten people to be present. When he did speak, he experienced tightness in his chest, difficulty concentrating (he said that his mind would "blank out"), sweating, a shaky voice, and a cottony dryness in his mouth. Once a court date was scheduled, Ted would begin worrying about it a month ahead of time, and it would be impossible to get off his mind. Although he had recently won an award for meritorious service, he avoided putting in for a promotion because it would mean increased courtroom appearances—or, as Ted put it, "torture."

He had lived with this problem for twenty years, never disclosing it to a soul. Even his wife was in the dark. Ted believed that his career would be derailed even more seriously if he revealed this problem to his boss. If it was ever exposed that he was visiting a "shrink," he expected the humiliation of being asked to turn in his weapon and take a desk job—all because of public speaking anxiety! We talked about some options for treatment, and Ted said he would think about them. But he never returned to pursue treatment.

The consequences Ted feared, should his boss have found out about his seeking help, might very well have been realistic. Although society has come a long way toward acceptance, severe stigma remains for even the mildest emotional disorders. The stigma seems stronger for men and strongest in those circles where machismo reigns supreme. Ironically, those who are likely to suffer the most shame from having a social anxiety problem are also likely to suffer the most stigma from getting the treatment they need. Fortunately, things are gradually changing for the better as the public becomes better informed about the facts of these disorders and their treatment.

TREMBLING, FEAR AND VIDEOTAPE

We have all had our share of social anxiety experiences. What stands out for me (F.S.) was one of my first appearances on a television talk show as an "expert" on anxiety. I had been invited to appear along with Jerilyn Ross, president of the Anxiety Disorder Association of

America, and two patients from our clinic. Getting the opportunity to be on TV was exciting. I knew my family and friends would get a kick out of seeing me, I would have the opportunity to get the word out to sufferers in the community, and the exposure would bring needed volunteers into our clinic's research program. Being recognized as an expert also made me feel successful and appreciated, even important.

We had some time to wait backstage before the videotaping, so I chatted with our patients, one of whom was a woman I had treated for social phobia. Our clinic is periodically the subject of media reports, but I'm always amazed when a patient with social phobia agrees to tell his or her story to the world. If I had recently recovered from social phobia, I might prefer to enjoy my new self-confidence quietly with friends and colleagues, but I admire the few who are eager to reach out publicly to help others in need.

I also talked with Jerilyn, whom I recognized as the leader of an organization that had done great work raising awareness of anxiety disorders in the community and among mental health professionals. We had never met before. She was very friendly, and also quite articulate, spirited, and photogenic. We recounted our prior experience with the media—my few brief interviews and her vast experience speaking around the country and hosting her own radio call-in show in Washington, D.C. I secretly felt a few twinges of unease. On the small screen, how could I possibly match up to this charismatic media personality? As I felt my anxiety rising, I reminded myself that I knew my stuff and that this was not a competition. I relaxed some and thought about the points I hoped to get across, but my competitive side did not completely disappear.

After we sat down on the set and the cameras started rolling, I was alarmed to feel my head start to tremble, as if a personal earthquake had begun with its epicenter at the base of my skull. The more I worried about it the worse it got. Would people notice? I assumed the pose of *The Thinker,* steadying my chin with my hand. (Is that what Rodin had in mind?) I *was* thinking—about what the audience would make of an anxiety disorder ''expert'' whose head shook with fear! ''Physician, heal thyself!'' And then the shaking disappeared as fast as it had come on. I got in my three sound bites, our patients were terrific telling their stories, and the show was over.

Later, when I watched the show on videotape, I discovered that my head, remarkably, appeared to have stayed in one place. I was critical of some other things I did (too much hand gesturing and looking too serious), but I felt relieved overall and chalked it up to experience.

Better yet, I made a note of my misperception and planned to use this experience to better help my patients. When the source of social anxiety is an actual misperception of how you appear to others, watching a videotape of yourself can be therapeutic, and this is sometimes useful as a self-help technique or to incorporate in psychotherapy.

4

PEOPLE ANXIOUS WITH PEOPLE

There is that destroyeth his own soul through bashfulness.

Apocrypha, Ecclesiasticus 20:22

Whereas fear of public speaking usually occurs in only a narrow slice of all the social situations a person encounters, the fears that accompany generalized social phobia pervade most aspects of a sufferer's life. In terms of overall impact, this form of social phobia can be the most devastating.

JACKIE

Jackie was a twenty-six-year-old single woman who said she was coming to see me (F.S.) as a last resort. Although she was strikingly attractive and well dressed, she appeared bashful, intermittently glancing up and then looking at the floor while she spoke softly. Her shyness dated back as far as she could remember, but more severe anxiety in nearly all social situations had become a problem for her at about age sixteen.

Nowadays it didn't take much to make her self-conscious and anxious. Spotting an acquaintance on the street caused her to worry she wouldn't say "the right thing," so she would try to avoid the person. Then she would fear that the person had noticed her avoidance and assumed she was unfriendly, and she would put herself down for

28

being socially inept. Going to parties was a struggle. She would get nauseous beforehand, worrying that she would embarrass herself by stumbling over words and that her friends would find her boring.

Jackie had noticed that alcohol often relieved her anxiety at parties, so she began to drink two to five shots of vodka *before* going to a party. Without drinking, she felt unable to attend. She considered the alcohol to be her "medication," but she was disgusted by her need for it and suffered hangovers afterward. She also realized that she could easily become more seriously addicted if she allowed herself to rely on it more regularly.

Dating was another troubling situation because she was convinced that no desirable man would want a woman who was so paralyzed by anxiety. Jackie's attractiveness, intelligence, and other assets didn't count for much in her mind, and she believed that normal people would feel no anxiety before a first date. She had dated some, self-medicating with alcohol before each date, but she hadn't been able to enjoy herself due to her fears. Jackie always managed to sever relationships after a few dates, when she feared she would be unable to continue to conceal her anxiety problem.

Jackie had done well in school and moved on to a job as an administrator in a large company. She was doing okay at work, but she knew she could do much better if she could only overcome her fear of speaking up at meetings and become more comfortable talking with her colleagues. Jackie wasn't clinically depressed, but she was demoralized, feeling that her true self was locked up by inhibitions.

As is the case for many people with generalized social fears, Jackie felt unable to put her finger on a particular reason why she should have developed these problems. Both of her parents were high achievers who tended to be demanding, even harsh at times, but they were never abusive. And her older sister had grown up with the same set of parents and had no problems with anxiety. There had been no unusual humiliations in her past that might explain her fears.

It also wasn't as if she had never sought help for these problems. In three years of individual psychotherapy, Jackie had learned some interesting things about the way she related to her family and subsequently improved her relationship with her mother, but her social problems were unchanged. Another therapist had misdiagnosed her condition as panic disorder and attempted to treat symptoms such as hyperventilation and avoiding anonymous crowds, although Jackie had neither problem. She had tried several medications with only modest results, and she felt they were not worth the hassle.

Although Jackie was feeling discouraged at this point, I remained optimistic. Jackie's problems fell squarely into the realm of general-ized social phobia. We had available several good treatment options that she had never before tried, using either medication or psychother-apy directed at her social phobia.

One real concern was Jackie's alcohol use. It is quite the norm, of course, for people to use alcohol to relieve social tension and loosen up at parties. However, once people with severe social anxiety learn that alcohol helps temporarily, it can quickly seem to become a neces-sity. Some people go on to develop problems due to their drinking, and they become alcoholics. Then they face another quagmire: Their social anxiety interferes with their ability to participate in alcoholism treatment groups such as Alcoholics Anonymous. At the same time, alcohol abuse clouds their ability to make use of psychotherapy and makes the use of certain medications for social phobia unsafe.

I recommended that Jackie enter a short-term specialized group therapy for social phobia, a treatment we will discuss further in chap-ter 18. In such a group she would have an opportunity to learn some techniques for recognizing and changing the irrational parts of her fears. The group setting would be ideal for getting honest feedback from supportive people who had experienced similar problems, and it would allow her to practice becoming gradually more assertive in a "safe" place. With her assets of intelligence, attractiveness, and a strong desire to change, I believed she was an excellent candidate to do well in such a group. She did not agree.

Jackie told me that she was through with therapy, that it had not helped before, and that she could never admit her fears to any group, no matter how supportive. She would not be budged. We turned to discussion of the several types of medication that recently have been shown to be helpful for social phobia. Jackie agreed to forgo alcohol, as she had been able to do temporarily while taking medicine in the recent past, in order to give the new medicine a try.

Two weeks after starting Paxil, Jackie began to notice some bene-fits. She was definitely more relaxed with people, and she was even able to enjoy certain social situations for the first time in a long while. She had felt a little nausea for a few days, and she wasn't sleeping as soundly as usual, but these side effects were tolerable for her. As we continued to monitor her progress over the next couple of months, her improvement became obvious—and not just to Jackie. Her parents commented that she seemed more confident. She'd enjoyed having a string of three dates in one week, and her boss had appreciated her increased participation in meetings.

After that initial dramatic improvement, in the next few weeks

Jackie experienced some reemergence of her old fears, which we talked over in our follow-up sessions. Over the following months she gained more consistent mastery over the fears, and she gradually became more and more comfortable in most of the activities that she had been avoiding for so long. She still considered herself to be shy, but it no longer interfered with her life.

5

FEAR OF EATING AND DRINKING IN PUBLIC

A woman should never be seen eating or drinking unless it be lobster salad and Champagne, the only true feminine & becoming viands.

Lord Byron, 1812

Sharing food with another human being is an intimate act that should not be indulged in lightly.

M. F. K. Fisher, 1949

For some people, a problem bigger than social conversation itself is what occurs around and between the conversation—such as eating and drinking. If you think about how important the sharing of food is to the survival of a pride of lions, or was to the survival of our own human ancestors; or even if you just consider how many etiquette books have been written to relieve uncertainty about incorrect table manners, you will realize that the dinner table is not such an unusual place to become anxious.

THE WOMAN WHO FEARED EATING AND AVOIDED DATING

Carla was a thirty-eight-year-old secretary who recalled that as a teenager she had been somewhat self-conscious and quiet. She had always hated being the focus of attention, preferring to fade into the background. Although others considered her attractive, she was usually dissatisfied with her appearance in small ways. None of these traits had ever caused her serious problems, however. She married her high school sweetheart, had a bunch of close friends, raised two children, and did well on her job.

The roof gradually caved in on Carla as her husband's drinking and unfaithful behavior increased over the years. Although she eventually no longer loved her husband, she had at first put up with his bad behavior for the sake of the kids and later because she dreaded the thought of being on her own. After years of urging from her friends and family, she had gotten a divorce and tried to move on with her life.

A couple of years after her divorce she finally agreed to let a friend set her up on a date. Her anxiety began to build, however, as soon as the date had been arranged. She hadn't dated since high school, and even then she'd had little experience. All the rules had changed, and she did not know how to act. She felt too old to be dating, and she felt unattractive.

Her date picked her up and they went to a restaurant that was too formal and expensive for Carla's tastes. The man turned out to be very quiet and intently focused on her, which made Carla even more uncomfortable. When her dinner arrived, the thought popped into Carla's head that the linguini on her plate looked huge in relationship to the size of her mouth. Carla had always felt self-conscious eating in front of strangers, but she began to focus on eating strategies as she never had before, as if she were a mover planning to deliver a huge sofa through a small doorway. There was the old technique of swirling the linguini on a fork supported by a spoon, but her husband had often teased her about ending up with a forkful too large to fit into her mouth. "That jerk," she thought. Cutting the pasta into small pieces would be safer, but it might seem weird to her date. He asked her if she was okay, if her food was all right. Carla made up a story that she had been feeling a little queasy all day, and she excused herself to the ladies' room.

She returned, still nervous, to her rapidly cooling linguini, which she managed to eat by bracing her fork with two hands to steady her trembling. To avoid spilling her glass of water, Carla brought her mouth down to the glass. She improvised to her date that as a kid she had fooled around with drinking from a cup while it was on the table. Her date looked skeptical, and she felt like an idiot.

The next day, she was surprised to find her nervousness returning suddenly in the lunchroom at work. Again she worried that her shaky hands would embarrass her, and she feared that everybody would recognize that she was falling apart. Bewildered by these experiences, Carla vowed to avoid dining out until her fears of trembling subsided. Eating at home was not a problem, but Carla had never realized how many opportunities she had to eat with others. She declined a breakfast meeting, literally wishing to avoid egg on her face. She avoided the lunchroom at work, left the wedding of a friend before the reception, and tried to avoid dates that included eating meals together. Four months later, when she still felt stymied, she accepted a friend's suggestion that she consult a therapist.

Carla entered a brief therapy group for people with social phobia. Together with her therapist, she set a goal to use the group to experiment with eating in front of others as a stepping-stone to eating with others in the real world. After a few sessions of reviewing her problems and learning some techniques to cope with her anxiety, she was ready to practice some new behavior.

Her therapist helped arrange a role play with another group member acting the role of a coworker. Carla's first goal was to drink a glass of water in front of her "coworker" without excusing herself from the room, while continuing to carry on a conversation with him in between sips. Afterward, the group reviewed how she had done. Although she had succeeded in her goal, Carla was disappointed that her hand had been a bit shaky. Group members reported that her tremor was barely noticeable.

Over a few months, Carla worked her way through an obstacle course of increasingly difficult foods and simulated social situations. She gradually gained confidence in both her eating and her social relationships, and she transferred her progress to some real-life situations through practice outside of the group. The culmination of her recovery was a small party with some of the friends she had made in the group. The *pièce de résistance?* Linguini, of course.

DAVE—WEDDING JITTERS, LITERALLY

Sometimes eating or drinking fears crop up only in particularly stressful situations. A college friend of mine (F.S.) was looking forward to getting married. A week before the wedding, he seemed happy, was looking forward to his new life with his bride, and was free of the common prewedding jitters. As we talked about the wedding plans over dinner, however, he confided that he was worrying about one thing—that his hand would tremble during the wedding ceremony, which called for him to hold a glass of wine as he took his vows. He feared he would spill the wine and embarrass himself in front of the people he most cared about.

Even I was a bit surprised. Dave was a community activist who had given many talks to groups. He was successful and well respected. I had never thought of him as a nervous person. In fact, *mellow* is a word that comes to mind in describing him. On the other hand, I'm never really surprised to hear about some performance anxiety, because it is everywhere one least expects it.

As we left the restaurant, I offered a true "curbside" consult, which was actually a one-session cognitive-behavioral therapy. First we laid out his fears: trembling; spilling wine; people noticing, assuming that he was nervous, and assuming that he was fearful of getting married and was perhaps troubled in other ways.

I questioned the accuracy of Dave's predictions and we came up with some rational responses to his fears: He wasn't actually sure he would tremble, because it had never happened before. Even if he did tremble, it was unlikely that he would actually spill wine in a noticeable way (to test this, I suggested that he "practice" to see how much trembling it took to spill a half-full glass of wine). Dave maintained the belief that people would notice if he did tremble, but he agreed that his family and friends were more likely to interpret this positively (that he was overcome with positive emotion) than negatively (that he was psychologically troubled). I suggested that Dave practice holding a cup of wine while imagining the wedding scene and coping with his fears using the new responses he had developed.

After all that, at the wedding itself, I forgot to notice how Dave did at holding the wine. (Perhaps I was too concerned about my own responsibilities in the ceremony.) On the reception line, however, Dave informed me that the plan had worked. He had practiced only once, but the idea that others would accept his tremor gave him confidence. The results were no tremor, no spillage, and more wine to drink.

6

FEARS OF BLUSHING AND SWEATING

There's a blush for won't, and a blush for shan't,
And a blush for having done it.
There's a blush for thought and a blush for naught,
And a blush for just begun it.

John Keats (1795–1821)

While fears of eating or drinking in public are most commonly related to concerns about trembling, other physical sensations of social anxiety can be major troublemakers. Two of the most common are blushing and sweating.

ANNE, THE BLUSHER

Anne appeared to be one of those charmed people who exist only on television—twentysomething, intelligent, in a great relationship, with a solid job in the publishing field, outgoing, close to her loving family. There seemed to be no stopping her success. But then the blushing started.

She was sitting in her boss's office, feeling just a bit tense about a report she had been rushing to complete, when she suddenly felt hot and flushed, got extremely self-conscious, and wanted to get out of the room. Her boss noticed that something was wrong, and after the meeting he inquired if Anne was okay. Anne dismissed the incident as a fluke and went on with her life. Six months later it happened again, however, and then it began to occur regularly in meetings, in situations where she had to deal with authority figures, and even in casual social conversations.

Anne noticed that during each episode the skin on her face, neck, and chest would become red and blotchy, her palms would sweat, and her heart would flutter. She felt as if her body were out of control, and she feared that others would think she was nuts. Afterward she would feel confused and depressed by her lack of control of these symptoms.

There was no rational reason for her to be panicking. In fact, her company was delighted with her overall performance. At a reception, her boss announced that Anne was the surprise recipient of an award. Suddenly she found herself at the podium in front of two hundred people. Her face was burning and she felt humiliated and unable to enjoy the honor at all. Somehow she managed to make a brief speech, for which people complimented her afterward. She was amazed she had been able to speak at all, but that didn't diminish her pain.

She had tried general psychotherapy, but talking about her life experiences didn't help. She began to avoid work presentations, then parties and other social events. To partially conceal her blushes, Anne developed a signature outfit, wearing blouses with buttoned-up collars year-round. Nothing seemed to help. Even routine activities such as returning goods to a store, visiting a medical doctor, or getting a haircut became embarrassing ordeals.

Anne contemplated interviewing for other jobs, but this just caused her anxiety levels to rise again. She found herself unable to enjoy anything, low in energy, crying daily, and consistently feeling hopeless. She had become seriously depressed on top of her anxiety.

When Anne came in for treatment, we decided to try a combination of group therapy and a medication with both antidepressant and anti-anxiety effects to treat most rapidly and effectively her symptoms of social phobia and depression. Within a few weeks she noticed clear improvement in her mood. Anne's first session in the social phobia group was an eye-opener—she never imagined that other normal-looking people could be going through similar problems. It was a huge relief to talk to people who understood. When she expressed aloud her fear that people who saw her blush would think she was crazy, it suddenly sounded ridiculous to her. Over several months of medication and therapy, her progress was gradual but steady. Her symptoms decreased tremendously, and she learned to make peace with the minor blushing that remained.

Blushing is an interesting anxiety symptom because it is so connected with the emotion of embarrassment. Charles Darwin was intrigued by blushing, and much of his commentary on the subject from 1870 still holds true. He noted that unlike laughing or frowning, a blush cannot be brought on voluntarily, and he recognized that it "is not the simple act of reflecting on our own appearance, but the thinking what others think of us, which excites a blush."

As a naturalist, Darwin pursued blushing with the same curiosity and powers of observation he used to study the behavior of animals, although he was limited by the bounds of Victorian propriety:

> I was desirous to learn how far down the body blushes extend . . . [a physician] who necessarily has frequent opportunities for observation, has kindly attended to this point for me during two or three years. He finds that with women who blush intensely on the face, ears, and nape of neck, the blush does not commonly extend any lower down the body. It is rare to see it as low down as the collar-bones and shoulder-blades. . . . Nevertheless Sir J. Paget informs me that he has lately heard of a case, on which he can fully rely, in which a little girl, shocked by what she imagined to be an act of indelicacy, blushed all over her abdomen and the upper parts of her legs. Moreau also relates, on the authority of a celebrated painter, that the chest, shoulders, arms, and whole body of a girl, who unwillingly consented to serve as a model, reddened when she was first divested of her clothes.

SWEATING IT OUT—VANCE

While sweating may not be quite the same hallmark of embarrassment as blushing, it can be an equally troubling symptom of social anxiety, as the deodorant industry has profitably noted.

Vance had often felt baffled by the different sides of his personality. On the one hand, he was solid and successful—a construction foreman, happily married with three children, and a good storyteller at parties. He had even been the popular captain of his high school football team. On the other hand, he was a self-conscious worrier who felt he could lose his job at any moment due to periods of obsessive fear of trembling and sweating in public.

Vance remembered fearing that his hands would shake as far back as when he was an altar boy in childhood, painfully enduring the scrutiny of the congregation. For a while during high school Vance had feared that people would notice him trembling when he signed his name, so he simplified his signature to get it over with more quickly. Vance also felt self-conscious during physical examinations, and when his blood pressure reading was strangely elevated, his doctor had diagnosed "white coat hypertension" and told him to take readings at home when nobody was scrutinizing him. Those readings were all normal.

These troubles paled in comparison, however, to Vance's latest scourge, sweating. He had always tended to sweat a lot, but when he was promoted to chief foreman, it suddenly got worse. One day he was in an argumentative meeting, and he noticed that unlike his adversary he was obviously perspiring. After the meeting, it occurred to him that sweating was a sign of weakness, that others would perceive him as having trouble handling the pressure. His job depended on the reputation he had built as a strong leader. The fears began to mount: If he were to lose his reputation he would be laid off, and at this stage of his life he'd have to find a new line of work. How would he cover the mortgage? How could he explain to his family that they'd have to cut out vacations, the kids' college plans . . .

Vance began thinking about his sweating problem at every meeting. The more he checked for sweat, the more he found it. He started wearing light-colored clothes that he thought were less likely to show sweat, but that wasn't enough. Later, in therapy, he confessed with embarrassment to having even experimented with using his wife's sanitary napkins as underarm shields. It was around this time that Vance decided to seek help to deal with his social anxiety.

The fears began to interfere directly with Vance's career. He would let his assistant handle important meetings if he was having a bad day or if the weather was too hot. He once interrupted a meeting to dash off to the men's room to towel himself dry surreptitiously. His career plans seemed to be evaporating while his perspiration would not.

Seeing that Vance was at a loss, his internist gave him an antidepressant to try, but Vance gave up on the drug when it didn't work after only a few days. His doctor had not mentioned that the medication might take weeks to work, and he did not follow up on Vance's results. A psychiatrist recommended a different antidepressant that had been shown to sometimes help social phobia symptoms, but for Vance it had the side effect of increased sweating, of all things, so he stopped taking it. Another therapist tried an approach that is often useful for social phobia, helping Vance to set some behavioral goals, such as purposely revealing his sweating problem to others. The therapist hoped this might allow Vance to recognize that his fears of devastating criticism were unfounded. Vance felt that his coworkers would never understand and that his job was on the line, however, so he was unwilling to pursue a course that seemed so risky.

After considering a few options, including another try at a more gradual behavioral therapy, Vance chose to try again to manage his problem with medication. The first medicine we tried, Klonopin, did reduce the sweating significantly, but he felt it made him a bit tired, taking a needed edge off his ability to perform at his peak. He then switched to Inderal, a medicine of another class that rarely affects mental sharpness, and this time the results were better. He would take the medicine before an important meeting, and just as he would expect to start sweating . . . it wouldn't happen. His confidence slowly came back. After a year he gradually discontinued using the medicine and found it had gotten him over the hump.

While Vance's phobia is "in remission" and he is no longer worried about embarrassing himself, he is not truly cured of his fears. Vance believes that if the sweating worsens for some reason in the future, he will need to go back on the medicine to handle it. We have talked about pursuing cognitive-behavioral therapy to see if he might overcome his fears more completely. At the moment, however, Vance prefers to leave well enough alone, and he continues to carry a couple of aging Inderal pills in his pocket . . . just in case.

7

DATING ANXIETY

There is no reason for the young man to be self-conscious in the presence of ladies. A little will power and a little sincere effort will banish this fault forever.

Lillian Eichler, *Book of Etiquette*, 1922

If overcoming fears of dating was as easy as Lillian Eichler once suggested in her *Book of Etiquette,* we could skip this section entirely. Unfortunately, for many people suffering persistent fears of dating, the well-meaning but simplistic advice they receive simply is not effective. Fortunately, there is another way.

JERRY

At first glance, Jerry's life didn't look like that of someone with a generalized social phobia. He was a successful graduate student in a prestigious computer science program, had good friends, appeared poised, had worked summers as a salesman, and even had performed onstage in a variety of singing groups. His problem was dating. While he had been on a number of first dates, they never seemed to lead to anything resembling a relationship.

It became clear, however, that Jerry had been struggling against social phobias his whole life. He had won most of the battles, or at least played them to a respectable draw. After a carefree early childhood, Jerry remembered gradually becoming concerned about how he

41

compared to other kids around the fifth grade. He realized that his clothes weren't "cool" and that he was a bit uncoordinated, so he started paying more attention to his appearance, and he worked harder to achieve success in sports. Still, he worried about how others would judge him.

Despite these fears, he continued to excel in school. He would speak up in class when he was sure he had a great idea, although teachers complained that he didn't speak up enough. He was a good singer in the high school chorus, although he never did as well as his teacher expected in auditions for all-state chorus. Jerry always had a few good friends and many acquaintances, but he worried a great deal about being liked. He feared that in his efforts to please others, he could be so agreeable and chameleonlike that people would find him dull. None of these limitations, however, would have ever led him to seek psychiatric help.

And then there were girls. As a teen, Jerry became interested in them. He liked to look at them, and he imagined dating, kissing, making love. But while he had female friends, he didn't dare date. Looking back on it, he realized that he had burdened himself with the demand that a prospective date be perfect. He recognized that one obstacle to this goal was that a perfect woman would probably reject him. Jerry would have been willing to settle for a less than perfect woman if he didn't fear devastating criticism and taunting from his male friends, who seemed to love to ridicule some of the girls he secretly admired.

Jerry suffered silently throughout high school. As his fears persisted, they grew more troubling. He worried about becoming a misfit, and he imagined a tortured lifetime without sex. He also wondered if people assumed he was gay, and he wondered if he *was* gay, despite his exclusive attraction to women.

One day a favorite teacher asked Jerry to stop by after class. The teacher passed on a bit of news: It so happened that a rather attractive classmate had mentioned her admiration for Jerry and her hope that he would ask her out. Jerry was pleased by the interest and embarrassed by how he'd found out, but he wasn't about to miss another opportunity. He asked her out and they had a typically awkward first date. Afterward Jerry was self-critical of his awkwardness but immensely relieved that he had broken the barrier of his avoidance.

In college Jerry felt less pressure to impress a clique of peers, and he was able to date some women. But a new layer of social phobic problems emerged: How to move from small talk to more revealing personal talk without inviting criticism from a date? How to move from being a gentleman to being a prospective lover without demeaning a woman by seeming too interested in sex? The result of all this cogitating was neither fun nor intimate relationships.

Since high school Jerry had wondered about seeking professional help for his problem. He assumed, however, that a person had to be quite mad to see a psychiatrist. The very act of doing so would be humiliating and impossible to reveal to his parents. What if a classmate found out? And would a therapist take his problem seriously?

So when Jerry finally decided to seek counseling while in graduate school, it was an emotionally wrenching and significant move. In fact, Jerry's decision to put himself on the line by seeking therapy reflected his readiness to take some chances and to confront his fears. More than anything specific that happened in his traditional psychotherapy, it was this readiness that led to some changes in his life. What did happen in therapy was that Jerry got the chance to practice revealing himself in a nonjudgmental setting. The more we looked over his life, the more it became clear to Jerry that he had more to lose by avoiding all risks than by putting himself on the line. He had been discounting his good qualities and magnifying the risks of just being himself. As he began to reveal more of himself in relationships, contrary to his fears, women seemed to like him more. Over time, he built up confidence and moved on with his life.

III

SOCIAL ANXIETY'S CAUSES: BODY, MIND, AND SOCIETY

8

WHAT GOOD IS SOCIAL ANXIETY?

Man is the only animal that blushes—or needs to.

Mark Twain, 1897

Although the irrational fears of embarrassment experienced by Harry and others with social phobia may seem exceptional, milder concerns about embarrassment are universal. Almost everyone has experienced some nervousness about approaching an authority figure or meeting somebody who is particularly attractive. Why are most of us so susceptible to social anxiety? Prior experiences of extreme humiliation might explain the fearfulness of some people, but they aren't common enough to account for the widespread vulnerability of our species to social anxiety. To explore the origins of this anxiety, we must go beyond the life experiences of an individual and consider the natural history of social fears over the whole of human evolution.

THE FORCES OF EVOLUTION

The forces of evolution tend to preserve features that enhance the survival of a species. Nature is full of behaviors that take their toll on the individual but persist over many generations because they benefit the species as a whole. Take the worker bee, who gives his all for the sake of the queen, or the mother hen who guards her eggs with

her life. Evolution may look kindly on certain characteristics and behaviors, even if they have disadvantages for the individual.

The forces of evolution are also conservative. Once a feature that
offers survival value has evolved, it tends to stick around, even if it
is no longer essential. For example, fingernails are nice to have, but
they hardly seem essential to survival. Their purpose can be better
appreciated, however, if we think of them as remnants of the claws
that were crucial to the survival of the lower animals from which
humans evolved. Although claws are not essential to human survival,
nature does not discard them.

We can use these two principles of evolution to examine common
human phobias. From this perspective, a phobia, although harmful to
the individual sufferer, might have some advantage for the survival
of the species. Such survival value may be clearer if we examine how
phobia behavior may have operated in our ancestors. The Swedish
psychologist Arne Öhman has used these principles to develop a pro-
vocative theory of social phobia. His theory, which we review below,
explains the evolution of social phobia by contrasting it with the
evolution of a simpler phobia—fear of animals.

ANCIENT FEARS, PRESERVED

The tendency to fear dangerous animals is one trait with obvious
survival value for both the individual and the human species. Fear of
animals, however, can also be excessive. When a person's fear of a
particular species, such as fear of dogs or fear of spiders, is severe
and irrational, it is considered a phobia. Why should such irrational
fears exist?

Through the millennia, those individuals among our human and
prehuman ancestors who were able to avoid dangerous predators (such
as lions) were less likely to be eaten by them. These individuals were,
therefore, more likely to live long enough to produce offspring.
Through this process of survival of the fittest, nature tended to select
individuals who were best able to detect dangerous animals and to
respond appropriately (for example, by fighting or by fleeing). Fear
of animals, therefore, is likely to have been shaped by the forces
of evolution.

In assessing the danger of predators, our ancestors could make two
types of errors, each with very different results. Our first caveman is a
nervous guy who generally fears animals much more than the average
caveman. He startles in response to a suspicious noise that he assumes
is a lion, only to discover that the noise was just the wind rustling

some leaves. His startle reaction to the "nonthreat" wastes some energy, but he suffers no serious consequences.

Being a nervous type, our caveman continues to believe that the next noise could be a real lion. His mellow cavemate, however, saunters off into the bush chuckling over his neighbor's misery, ignores lion tracks on his trail, and becomes lunch. The point is that when a threat from predators is uncertain, it is adaptive for a person to be biased in favor of overreacting. This adaptive advantage for individuals who sometimes overreact offers a mechanism for survival of persons with phobias of animals.

PREPARED FOR FEAR

For much of the evolutionary history of mammals, reptiles were among the most dangerous predators, and Öhman notes that their role as the incarnation of Evil has lived on in folktales of dragons (and in modern tales from *Godzilla* to *Jurassic Park,* we might add). It is, therefore, not surprising that fear is easily triggered in mammals by such cues as reptile-like pairs of forward-looking eyes or the sensation of slimy skin. In fact, fear of snakes is particularly easy for humans and monkeys to acquire and difficult for them to overcome.

The power of fear of snakes was demonstrated by the following experiment by psychologist Susan Mineka. Laboratory-reared rhesus monkeys, which did not fear snakes and had never actually seen one, rapidly developed an intense fear of snakes after they watched a brief videotape of a wild-reared monkey responding fearfully to a toy snake. Animals from another group of laboratory-raised monkeys, which had also never seen rabbits, were then shown the identical videotape spliced so that the "actor" monkey appeared to be responding fearfully to a toy rabbit. However, after watching the second video the monkeys developed no fear of rabbits. It was far easier for these inexperienced monkeys to develop a fear of snakes than to develop a fear of rabbits.

The experiment suggests that the brain of a mammal is not a blank slate when it comes to fear, but instead, as psychologist Martin Seligman has theorized, the infant's brain comes "prepared" to readily acquire certain useful types of fear. Other obviously protective and adaptive fears, which commonly appear in an extreme form as phobias, include fear of heights and fear of the dark.

Because young animals are most vulnerable to predators, Öhman suggested that the pressures of natural selection would particularly favor survival of young animals that effectively detect and respond to predators. For example, a young monkey that ran to its mother whenever there was an unexpected noise would be more likely to survive than a bold young monkey who went off to explore every unexpected noise. These surviving animals would pass on to their offspring the trait of being good at detecting predators during youth. Humans, of course, do tend to be most fearful of animals in childhood. Similarly, phobias of animals, such as snakes, spiders, or dogs, are most common in childhood and begin at an earlier age than most other types of common phobias.

ALL ANXIETY IS NOT ALIKE

Unlike this relatively straightforward explanation for the evolution of animal phobias, the reasons why social phobia should exist are not so apparent. Social anxiety does not seem to directly protect survival. The person with social phobia, after all, fears not an ancestral predator but a member of his own species. Often, that member of the same species is not even dangerous, but instead may be particularly attractive and important to the phobic person. Instead of fearing bodily harm, as does the animal phobic, the person with social phobia usually fears embarrassment or humiliation. Social phobia seem unlikely to have developed from the same sources as animal phobias.

Öhman noted that differences in the physical symptoms of social fear and fear of dangerous animals further suggest that these fears have evolved separately. The physiological response to physical danger has been called the "fight-or-flight" response. This response speeds up the heart rate and shunts blood from the digestive tract, where it is not needed at the moment, to the muscles of the extremities. These changes serve to prepare one's body to counterattack or to flee to safety. The fight-or-flight response is triggered by predators and other dangers, and it is likely to have contributed to the survival of our ancestors.

While the fight-or-flight response is sometimes a feature of social anxiety (especially public performance anxiety), the social anxiety response may also include different symptoms—such as blushing, averting the gaze from others, or displaying a sheepish grin. (These specialized appeasement behaviors, we shall see, offer clues to the evolutionary purpose that social anxiety serves.) Social phobia also differs from the other phobias in that it tends be more prevalent in the adolescent years, instead of in early childhood. This suggests that social fears may have evolved to deal with challenges that are greatest during adolescence, such as establishing one's own place in society and finding a mate.

To understand the evolutionary origins of social phobia, therefore, we need to shift our focus away from the issue of maximizing chances of individual survival. By its very nature, social anxiety can best enhance survival in another way, through social means. Our ability to live in stable social groups, such as extended families and clans, has been crucial to the survival of the human race. Social groups provided a safe setting for the lengthy process of rearing human offspring, and social cooperation and division of labor gave us an edge in hunting, despite our limited physical abilities. The social systems of humans and our primate ancestors are so crucial to the survival of our species that they must have been shaped along the way by natural selection.

A Summary of Öhman's Evolutionary Theory of Social Phobia

	FEAR OF PREDATORS	SOCIAL FEARS
Evolutionary origin of fear	more ancient	less ancient
Function of the fear	protects the individual	stabilizes the group
What/who is feared	another species	member of same species
Type of fear response	only fight-or-flight	also appeasement behaviors
Age of peak fear	early childhood	adolescence
Associated human disorder	animal phobias	social phobias

RANK HAS ITS PRIVILEGE

If Öhman's theory is correct, and social concern or anxiety does have survival value for humans, similar phenomena should be present in other primate species that live in social groups. In other words, monkeys and other species related to our ancestors should show some form of social anxiety. And scientists have indeed found these possible roots of human social anxiety in the behaviors that preserve social groups among animals.

Such behaviors, ranging from submissiveness and social fear behavior at one end to dominance and aggressive behavior at the other end, often emerge in encounters between animals of the same species. It is known as social ranking behavior. These ranking encounters, while antagonistic, are often highly ritualized, and in higher mammals they rarely lead to serious injuries. For example, sheep fight each other by first backing off, then charging and butting heads. Their thick horned skulls protect against serious injury. Sheep never butt the flank of an unsuspecting opponent, although such an attack could be much more damaging. In group-living monkeys, ranking encounters result in a dominance hierarchy in which each animal holds a particular rank within its community.

The English psychologist Paul Gilbert has suggested that changes in the nature of social ranking behaviors over evolutionary history are important for understanding human social behavior. For reptiles and birds, rank determines which individual animal within a species will be able to breed in a particular territory. A pecking order emerges through a series of one-on-one confrontations between individuals. In these contests the animals may face each other, stand tall, and display ritualized head movements and dancelike behaviors. These behaviors allow each animal to size the other up—to figure out who is stronger or weaker. The weaker animal, based on this assessment, can choose to flee the territory and escape certain harm. Thus, the ability to display social rank and to assess another's social rank insures that stronger, healthier animals will be more likely to breed and to pass on their genes, and it allows weaker animals to flee to another territory, where they can get another chance to adapt more successfully.

THE POWER OF SUBMISSIVE BEHAVIOR

Species of monkeys and apes also exhibit ranking behaviors. Because they often live in large social groups, however, there are important differences in their needs. Animals that live solitary lives can flee a territory if they are defeated by a dominant member of their species. However, in species that benefit from living in social groups, fleeing the group may not be a viable option, so it now becomes important for a weaker individual to be able to "surrender" to a dominant animal.

In fact, there are a variety of nonverbal behaviors in monkeys and apes that convey the very message "I am submissive, and I will not challenge your authority." These behaviors emphasize a surrendering body posture by looking down, crouching, and bowing, which make the body look smaller and less threatening; lowering the chin; and turning away. The animal may also display fearful grins and emit whimpers and squeaks that signal distress. This body language bears a striking resemblance to some behavior in shy, embarrassed humans. Could socially anxious behavior in humans have an analogous role as a surrender signal? As further evidence of the profoundly communicative nature of this behavior in monkeys, some subordinate chimpanzees have been observed to actually reach out and move their opponents' faces so the opponents would see their submissive expression.

Gilbert notes further that species that have the ability to signal submission can maintain their dominance hierarchies via power or threat of harm, rather than by resorting to actual fights, which are more costly. And it is not only the leader who enforces such a hierarchy. In social groups of primates, such as chimpanzees, the lower-ranking animals take an active role in maintaining the hierarchy by recognizing the stronger individuals and submitting to them.

When animals contest the leadership of a hierarchy, the ranking becomes unstable. At such times low-ranking animals need to be vigilant (or perhaps "anxious") when around stronger animals of uncertain rank, to avoid even accidentally appearing to challenge their authority. When a hierarchy is stable and each individual "knows his place" relative to the others, overall levels of aggression may be quite low. In this way, social anxiety, avoidance, and submissiveness help stabilize the social group by preventing confrontations that could lead to violence and costly injuries.

SELF-CONSCIOUS CHIMPS

To maintain stable dominance hierarchies, individual monkeys and chimpanzees must have a remarkable awareness of their social rank in relationship to others. The level of self-consciousness of which chimpanzees are capable is evidenced by the following observation by the primatologist Frans DeWaal.

Chimps tend to be sexually promiscuous, but if a female and a low-ranking male wish to copulate, they must avoid being seen or heard by a "jealous" dominant male, who would otherwise break up the tryst. One adolescent female, Oor, had a habit of screaming particularly loudly during copulation, and as a result many of her surreptitious matings with low-ranking males were interrupted by dominant males who heard her scream. Eventually she learned to stifle her scream during the clandestine copulations, although she continued to vocalize freely when mating with the dominant male.

Had Oor learned a form of sexual modesty? We can surmise that she had some awareness of the implications of the rank of her sexual partners. Before assuming that sexual modesty occurs in nature, however, we might consider the alternative view stated by the French philosopher Denis Diderot in 1796: "The pleasures of love are followed by a weakness which puts one at the mercy of his enemies. That is the only natural thing about modesty; the rest is convention."

Even more sophisticated self-conscious behavior, such as trying to hide signs of social fear (recall, for example, the effort Harry made to conceal the shakiness of his hands from his audience while he made a toast), may not be unique to humans. DeWaal describes an old dominant male named Yeroen who was being challenged repeatedly by a younger chimp. Yeroen seemed to try to hide the signs of his uncertainty from his rival. After a conflict Yeroen kept an expressionless face until he was alone, and only then did he release a fearful grin and yelp. In another example, a chimp named Luit began to show a fearful grin when challenged, but immediately put his hand to his mouth and manually pressed his lips together. When the challenger was out of sight, Luit started grinning submissively and gave a soft distressed squeak. These males appear to have been suppressing and concealing their signs of fear and submission.

HUMAN COMPETITION AND COOPERATION

Like chimpanzees, we humans are highly aware of our social status relative to other persons (our position in the human dominance hierarchy). Even four-year-olds have been shown to reliably identify their own dominance ranking in relationship to nursery school classmates. We also generally prefer to have dominant status, again sharing this characteristic with chimps, who often put great effort into achieving the highest possible rank. Individuals who are lower in the hierarchy would be expected to generally experience more social anxiety, because they are at greater risk for being challenged by more dominant individuals.

Although social competition pervades our society, ranking by power is not the only way to look at human relationships. Human social groups are also cemented by the concern that individuals have for other members of the group, and by our ability to show and to receive affection. Over the course of evolution, people who were effective at cooperating and using group activities for hunting and defense had survival advantages. So natural selection may have favored the survival of individuals who were concerned about others. A by-product of natural selection, therefore, might be the existence of some individuals with too much of this good thing, meaning excessive concern about what others think. We can speculate that this is another way in which social phobia might have originated as an extreme form of a basically adaptive behavioral system.

Some social scientists have noted that rank tends to be a preoccupation of males (in both animals and humans), and that women traditionally have been more concerned about social cohesion and fostering the success of family members. Psychologist Jean Baker Miller has stated that women generally do not see relationships in terms of power or as "zero-sum games." Instead they are more cooperative and try to foster everyone's development as opposed to competing.

Linguist Deborah Tannen has noted that this difference in attention to rank is reflected in both the speech and the behavior of men and women. She offers the example of a couple who are lost on the road. Harold resists asking for directions. He views asking as a sign of weakness; to ask for directions would be a blow to his self-esteem. Sylvia, however, has no reservations about asking for help. To her, asking is not a matter of losing a competition; instead, it creates relationships and reinforces bonds between people.

Psychologist Gilbert maintains that one form of social anxiety occurs in people who focus too much on fears of losing rank (being humiliated), rather than on making positive social connections. A focus on rank may be advantageous in certain situations, such as when approaching a large stranger in a dark alley. In that situation, it may make sense to act nonthreatening in order to avoid attack. It doesn't help Jerry, however, who has social phobia, to think the same way when approaching a desirable (high-ranking) woman for a date. Dating, like many human social situations, calls for a more positive mode of interaction in which individuals seek the cooperation of others by being warm and engaging.

The distinction between the dominance system on the one hand, and the cooperation/attractiveness system on the other, is sometimes blurred, because attractiveness itself can contribute to dominance. As Gilbert has suggested, humans typically want the power to attract and hold the attention of others through admiration, love, respect, and understanding, rather than just power over territory or mating rights. We also want power to be bestowed on us voluntarily, rather than being forced. Harry wants his family and friends to appreciate his speech (thereby acknowledging his status at the wedding), but he sees no clear sign of the audience's reaction, and he fears that he is losing the audience's appreciation of him.

There is some evidence that chimps, like humans, may experience anxiety related to the loss of positive attention, not just to the fear of being attacked. For example, an animal that has just lost a ranking encounter will often go back to the dominant animal to demonstrate its submission and obtain reassurance by getting positive attention from the dominant animal. The primatologist Jane Goodall describes the case of old Flo, who lost a fight with the dominant or "alpha male" chimp Mike and then offered him submissive gestures. Mike responded by embracing and patting her until she stopped screaming. He then groomed her for ten minutes, after which Flo was so calm that she actually slept with her head almost on Mike's foot. Once the dominance status between them was clear, the two individual animals were able to interact affectionately.

HOW WE SHOW SUBMISSION

Even when humans experience social anxiety for uniquely human reasons, the way that anxiety is expressed in our physiology and our behavior shares much with our primate relatives. Gilbert points out that the evolutionary shift from lower animals' fears of physical attack by a dominant animal to human fears of loss of attractiveness has been gradual over history. The behaviors that occur during ranking encounters, such as submission gestures, have changed relatively little. It is, therefore, not surprising that the chimpanzee's lowered gaze, hunched-over posture, and sheepish grin communicate submission quite eloquently to an observing human.

But we also show some differences from our primate relatives in our physiological responses to social anxiety. One such difference is the phenomenon of social blushing, which Charles Darwin called "the most peculiar and the most human of all expressions." The blush has no proven biological function, although if social anxiety did evolve as a social signaling system, blushing could be nature's own red traffic light. Psychologist Mark Leary has speculated that blushing might serve to reduce undesired attention from others. In the context of an embarrassment reaction, a blush sends the message "I care about what you think of me. I am not a threat to you, so you do not need to prove your dominance over me or to attack me." The ability to send such messages would have carried important survival value.

One problem with this social traffic light theory is that in persons with dark complexions the signal may remain invisible. People of color do, however, get a similar increase of blood flow to the face when they are embarrassed. An alternative explanation is that blushing acts as an internal social warning system. The warmth of increased blood flow serves to call the embarrassed person's attention to his own face and to reinforce the fact that he is being scrutinized. Paying attention to one's face serves to increase self-consciousness, which in turn distracts a person from aggressive impulses and further intensifies appeasing behaviors, making clear to the other that he or she is not being challenged.

EVOLUTION AND ENVIRONMENT

If human social anxiety does have roots in an ancient evolutionary advantage to the species, what does this imply for understanding anxiety problems? One implication is that social concerns and anxieties are an integral and adaptive part of human nature. They are integral in the sense that the capacity for these social feelings and behaviors is built into our genes. They are adaptive in that a moderate level of social anxiety does appear to confer advantages for individuals as well as for society. For example, having some concern about how others will judge our performance helps motivate us to function at our best in such sophisticated variations of ranking activities as interviewing for a job or asking someone out on a date. An optimal level of anxiety helps mobilize energy and concentration for the task at hand to enhance performance. Likewise, a moderate level of anxiety and a healthy sense of embarrassment can inhibit foolhardy or potentially dangerous behavior, such as fighting with a boss after being chided for making an avoidable error.

In social relationships, a moderate level of shyness may be adaptive in attracting the curiosity of others. A gentle demeanor may put other shy people or children at ease, and it may even attract the opposite-type "dominant" individual. Many societies value such submissive behaviors as showing modesty about one's achievements, blushing, or expressing embarrassment about explicit sexual matters.

The human social anxiety system, like most biologically based systems, can be disordered in some individuals or can be maladaptive in certain environments or situations. Social phobia involves excessive and maladaptive social fears. Harry's anxiety about public speaking, if it had not become excessive, might have effectively motivated him to prepare his speech well and to concentrate on his delivery. In its excessive form, however, it had the capacity to detract from the quality of his performance. Like many human afflictions, social phobia is an example of our species's adaptive defenses taken to a destructive extreme.

Evolutionary biology suggests why social phobia might have come to exist in the human *species*, but it does not help us explain how social phobia occurs in any particular *individual*. A person could theoretically develop social phobia by genetic and/or several types of environmentally influenced routes.

Some individuals may be genetically prone to submissive behavior. "Ancient" submissive behaviors, such as averted gaze, that have been passed down from evolutionary ancestors in other species may be particularly influenced by inheritance. There is evidence for a substantial genetic contribution to social phobia, a topic we will discuss in chapter 9.

Environmental factors, including the influence of family and culture, can also play a crucial role in developing social phobia. Dominance status or attention-holding power is not fixed at birth in animals or persons. People can move up or down in rank over time, depending on their actions and their surroundings. We simultaneously hold different ranks in the different social groupings and activities in which we participate. For example, a brilliant but overweight scientist might command great respect and power in the environment of his laboratory, yet feel self-conscious and inferior when sunbathing at the beach.

PATHWAYS TO SOCIAL ANXIETY

We have already noted several possible pathways from evolution to social anxiety. First, individuals who generally feel inferior or subordinant to others (whatever the cause) will tend to be more threatened by social encounters. Second, people who tend to view social encounters as an opportunity to test their rank in the hierarchy (rather than as an opportunity to communicate and form bonds) also will be more prone to social anxiety. For example, Harry might have (consciously or unconsciously) interpreted his selection as best man to mean that the groom gave him a status above other guests. In viewing his selection as a ranking event in which he has "defeated" others and become "dominant," he also views himself as a target for attack if he doesn't prove worthy.

Although women tend to have less competitive attitudes, they are not free from concerns about how others perceive them. Women's fears may focus less on loss of their own rank, however, and more on loss of connectedness to and affection of others, loss of rank for their family or friends, or being seen by others as too dominant or aggressive. The same social sensitivity that may foster women's group-centered attitudes may account for the tendency of women to suffer from social anxiety more often than men.

For both sexes, it is notable that social phobia can also occur in people who otherwise seem "dominant." Social anxiety can occur when a person of any status fears *loss* of status or loss of love of another, or when a person fears that his or her status is not being perceived as desired, as Mark Leary has noted. Some other ways that concern about rank might lead to social anxiety are as follows:

1. Gain of social rank may trigger fears. For example, promotion to a job that requires leadership skills may uncover previously dormant social fears. Appearing too dominant can also generate embarrassment. For example, Susan is a modest person who felt anxious when her boss praised her in front of her coworkers. She was uncomfortable with holding that kind of higher status at work (her boss had singled *her* out for praise and had not praised her coworkers), and she also feared in the back of her mind that "dominant" colleagues who felt challenged might retaliate against her. She expressed this discomfort through blushing and trembling (anxiety symptoms that nonverbally signaled her submissive status), self-effacing comments (verbally signaling her submissive status), and self-sabotaging behavior like "forgetting" to attend the next meeting (encouraging others to take away her dominant status).

2. A person might generally care little about rank but be thrust into a situation where dominance is all-important (for example, a homemaker who in the process of a difficult divorce finds herself fighting for a settlement in court).

3. A person might misjudge his or her own relative rank. People with this problem might believe they are losing status even when they are not. In this scenario, Harry might have been incorrect in his belief that giving the toast with a shaky voice would lead everyone to think badly of him. A hypothetical poll taken later in the reception might have shown that 97 percent of the guests were instead moved by the touching emotion he conveyed through his voice.

4. A trait that had elevated a person's rank may have actually been lost; for example, when a "self-made" businessman loses his business.

5. Change in social surroundings may raise new social ranking concerns; for example, when a successful individual leaves home for another country where his ethnic background is widely ridiculed.

Finally, other evolutionary factors may also play a role in some forms of social phobia. Innate fears of forward-staring eyes, already discussed in terms of predator fears, could also contribute to some social phobias. Being stared at is anxiety-provoking for many species, causing chicks to freeze and monkeys to feel threatened. In certain circumstances, human gaze that is too direct or prolonged may also stimulate certain automatic pathways of fear.

In summary, theories of the role of evolution in social anxiety offer an intriguing perspective on human social fears and phobias. They hold some promise that further research into animals' social behaviors may provide useful animal models for understanding aspects of social phobia in humans. At the same time, evolutionary theories are compatible with theories that both genetics and environment influence the development of social phobia.

9

BIOLOGICAL UNDERPINNINGS

My own brain is to me the most unaccountable of machinery—always buzzing, humming, soaring roaring diving, and then buried in mud. And why?

Virginia Woolf, 1932

WHY BIOLOGY?

At first blush, biology might seem to have little to offer in helping us understand social anxiety and social phobia. We cannot measure a level of social phobia in the blood, as we can cholesterol. We cannot biopsy social phobia to determine if it is benign or malignant, as we can a tumor. Social phobia can seem to be all in the mind. Embarrassment seems to be caused by certain social situations, from acting onstage to attending a cocktail party, and we don't think of either Shakespeare or small talk as particularly biological.

Yet social anxiety and social phobia are also highly physical experiences that we experience partly through such bodily sensations as blushing and trembling. What makes the vessels in our cheeks fill with blood against our will, and what makes our muscle fibers contract out of sync? These sensations are grounded in the workings of multiple bodily systems. Even the typical thought patterns of fear of embarrassment must also exist physically in certain patterns of electrical and chemical activity in brain pathways. Our body and brain physiology, in turn, are partially determined by the genes we inherited from our parents. So biology, in many ways, has quite a bit to do with social anxiety.

The biological roots of social anxiety run deep through human history and beyond. We discussed in chapter 8 the evidence that social anxiety developed over the course of evolution. From an evolutionary perspective, therefore, social anxiety might be an unpleasant by-product of an otherwise valuable social awareness system. This system, which is built into the brain, causes humans and other social animals to compare their strength or power to that of others around them. It allows us to signal submission when we feel overmatched, thereby avoiding dangerous fights over social rights.

One of the evolutionary legacies of our ancestors, the biological "hardwiring" of our brains, has built-in strategies for dealing with social contacts. This hardwiring underlies all our complicated social rituals, from dating etiquette to asking the boss for a raise. Similarly, it is the foundation for our complicated psychological conflicts over how to deal with others—from our desire to dominate others versus our desire to be taken care of, and from our wish to be admired versus our fear of being rejected.

PATHWAYS TO ANXIETY

The control center of this action is the brain. From outside the body, information floods the senses continuously and is relayed to the brain to be sorted out. Based on this information, the brain determines whether we should pay attention—and, if so, to which particular incoming signals. In this way the brain acts like a doorman at an exclusive nightclub, selecting the socially important from among the riffraff. The brain picks out key pieces of social information, such as an angry face, from a bombardment of mostly irrelevant light waves, sound frequencies, chemical particles that we experience as smells and tastes, and physical touches that the senses detect and begin to process.

The brain is expert at recognizing incoming social signals and interpreting whether they suggest danger. Part of this processing is conscious (that is, we experience it as thinking), and it takes place primarily in the brain's cerebral cortex. Another faster part of this processing is outside of our awareness, or automatic. Automatic brain activity passes through a brain structure called the amygdala. A fear response, if it develops, gets communicated to the rest of the body in two important ways: hormone messengers such as adrenaline are released into the bloodstream; and electrochemical impulses travel along nerve pathways. These hormones and nerve signals reach "end organs," such as the heart or sweat glands, where they trigger physiological responses such as increased heart rate or sweating.

So the body's social anxiety response, once set off by the automatic pathways of the brain, travels a well-trodden path of nervous system activation. This results in a characteristic pattern of physiological changes: the activation of certain nerve pathways within the brain cortex is experienced as feelings and thoughts of social anxiety. The blood vessels in the face receive signals to let their walls relax, allowing them to fill with more blood. Nerve signals that normally put the brakes on the heart rate may lessen, allowing the heart to speed up.

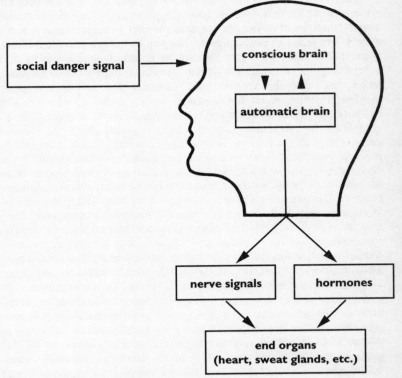

The brain has pathways for conscious and automatic processing of social danger signals.

As the automatic responses of body organs enter a person's conscious awareness, they are experienced as physical *symptoms* of social anxiety such as blushing (from the engorgement of blood vessels in the face), trembling (from the changes in muscle tone in the extremities and neck), and racing heart or palpitations (from changes in intensity, rate, and rhythm of heart muscle contractions). The awareness of these symptoms by the conscious brain may then lead to increased feelings of anxiety, embarrassment, or an urge to flee.

PERSONAL CHEMISTRY, PERSONAL FEARS

Up until now we have been discussing mechanisms that seem to be present in all humans—we all have the potential to experience social anxiety. Individual differences in susceptibility to social anxiety, however, might relate to differences at any step in the physiological chain. Some people may be hypersensitive to detecting social signals and interpreting them negatively—their ''antennae'' pick up ambiguous frowns, raised eyebrows, and body language that nobody else takes to mean anything much. Others may interpret social signals normally but have an overactive hormonal response to stressors, pumping adrenaline into the bloodstream at the slightest social threat. Or certain body organs might be especially easily activated, like a heart that is prone to palpitations or sweat glands that turn on like faucets. Some persons' brains may be particularly sensitive to what is going on in the rest of the body, so these people would be overly aware of minor sweating or trembling. There are many ways in which the unique biology of each individual might shape typical thought patterns, feelings, behaviors, and physical symptoms—all components of the anxiety response.

Just as the unique biology and chemistry of one's brain influences the way a person interacts with the outside world, events in the outside world can influence the chemistry of the brain. This seems especially true of experiences that occur repeatedly during childhood, while the brain is still developing most rapidly and growing the most new connections between nerve cells. Laboratory monkeys who grow up in groups without parents, and are thereby completely deprived of adequate mothering, show persistently higher levels of the brain neurotransmitter serotonin, which is a crucial chemical regulator of social interactions. These monkeys are persistently more timid in their social relationships than their normally raised peers.

Recent studies in humans have demonstrated that life experiences can alter the anxiety response system of the body. Both Holocaust survivors and combat veterans with posttraumatic stress disorder have been shown to produce lower-than-normal levels of the stress hormone cortisol. It is as if their experiences with trauma have "burned out" their bodies' ability to mount a normal physiological response to stress. MRI (magnetic resonance imaging) brain scans have shown the hippocampus area of the brains of Vietnam combat veterans with posttraumatic stress disorder actually to be smaller than normal, possibly a physical consequence of the psychological trauma of their war experiences.

If we speculate somewhat beyond the research data, other negative life experiences (for example, years of repeated put-downs or humiliations by a parent) could potentially lead to chemical and even structural abnormalities in the human brain. The changes induced by such persistent or extreme negative experiences may leave a person more vulnerable to severe anxiety in social or performance situations. It is possible that such a biological vulnerability could be corrected directly by medication, or alternatively could even be corrected by positive life experiences or successful psychotherapy.

The growing evidence of the two-way street that links biology and life experience has made it highly unlikely that complex phenomena like social anxiety will ultimately be explained as purely biological or purely psychological. So accepting a biological basis to our emotions in no way leads us to reject the influence of life experiences. In the past, members of the scientific community have often taken sides to debate whether nature (biology and genetics) or nurture (psychology and life experience) causes human problems. Today, these tired arguments are finally giving way to more sophisticated arguments over the complex ways in which biological tendencies *interact* with life experiences to shape who we become.

Our understanding of how the brain and nervous system function in social anxiety and other emotional processes is still very limited compared to our understanding of the functioning of other organs, such as the heart, liver, or kidneys. This is not surprising, given the complexity of the brain, with its more than 10 million highly interconnected nerve cells. The brain is also particularly difficult to study. It has no moving parts to observe. The brain's overall shape and size mean little, and even its microscopic structure yields only subtle clues into its function. Its patterns of electrical impulses and chemical messengers change from moment to moment, and any one type of chemical messenger molecule may deliver very different messages depending on where in the brain it is delivered. The brain's diversity rivals that of the human behavior it produces. Nevertheless, a number of ingenious experiments have begun to illuminate what was long considered an unknowable black box.

ALL IN THE FAMILY?

One approach to unmasking biological factors in social anxiety is to search for their origins in the genes. Genes are pieces of the inherited DNA blueprints, present in every cell of a body, that determine whether an organism will grow up to become a person or a fish—and that influence what kind of person or fish will result. Genes determine many physical features of individuals, but their role in human behavior and mental disorders has been less clear. The question of the extent to which genes influence a person's chances of developing social anxiety or social phobia can be answered through the study of families, and particularly through the study of twins.

If a tendency toward social anxiety is based on genes—that is, is biologically inherited—then social anxiety can be expected to run in families. Just as a pair of brothers are more likely than a pair of cousins to share the same eye color, genetically based behaviors should be more alike among relatives who are more closely related. Researchers Abby Fyer and Salvatore Mannuzza at Columbia University have studied the tendency of social anxiety to run in families. Their group interviewed family members (blood relations, including parents, siblings, and children) of patients with social phobia. These family members were compared to a control group, family members of volunteers who had never had social phobia or any mental disorder. Psychiatric evaluations of both groups of family members revealed that the rate of social phobia was three times higher in families of social phobia patients than in families of control group subjects (16 percent versus 5 percent). This suggests that social phobia does tend to run in families, to some extent.

A follow-up study divided the social phobia patients into those with generalized social phobia (who were generally shy and feared embarrassment in most social situations) and those who feared only a few types of social situations (such as public speaking or performing onstage). Only the generalized social phobia patients had a significantly higher rate of social phobia in their families. The families of these patients did not have an elevated rate of other psychiatric conditions, such as depression or schizophrenia.

The findings of the study show that the generalized subtype of social phobia (but probably not the performance or public speaking subtype) does run in families. They also demonstrate that a family member's higher risk of getting social phobia is not just part of a generally higher risk for getting any psychiatric disorder. In summary, a person with social phobia is more likely than chance to have other family members with the same problem. Other similar studies have supported this finding.

TWINS AND THE GENETICS OF SOCIAL PHOBIA

Showing that social phobia runs in families, however, does not prove whether this tendency is passed down to the next generation genetically (such as by one or several "social phobia genes") or environmentally (such as when children learn certain social behaviors by observing their parents). Studies of twins allow researchers to offer a more specific estimate of the relative contribution of genetic and environmental factors. Within families, persons with different relationships share different percentages of genetic heritage. For example, identical twins, who develop from a single sperm and egg, share 100 percent of their genes. Nonidentical (fraternal) twins share only 50 percent, however, as do any other pair of full siblings. If social phobia was a simple hereditary disorder, determined by inheritance of a single social phobia gene, then when one identical twin had social phobia, the other twin would always have it, too. In the language of genetics, they would be *concordant* for social phobia. Among fraternal twins, however, only 50 percent of pairs would be concordant for the disorder.

If social phobia was only *partially* hereditary (as most mental disorders, personality traits, and even some purely physical traits such as height appear to be), it would not be totally concordant in identical twins. It would, however, be *more* concordant in identical twins than in fraternal twins. On the other hand, if social phobia was purely determined by environment, then identical twins would be no more likely than fraternal twins to be alike in respect to having social phobia. Researchers have developed complex mathematical models to estimate how much of the similarity of a particular trait in a group of twins is due to genetics and how much is due to environment.

Psychiatrist Kenneth Kendler, a leader in applying these powerful new statistical tools to psychiatric disorders, reported a large twin study of social phobia at the Medical College of Virginia. Kendler studied more than two thousand pairs of female twins who were part of a research registry of twins in Virginia. When one member of an identical twin pair had social phobia, there was a 24 percent chance that the other member of the pair had it, too. The concordance rate for identical twins (24 percent) was higher than the rate for fraternal twins (15 percent). Using mathematical models, Kendler was able to estimate that genetic inheritance accounted for about 30 percent of the chance of developing social phobia, with environmental factors accounting for the remaining 70 percent. Other twin studies, using different definitions of social fears and different mathematical models, have estimated the genetic contribution at anywhere from 22 percent to 50 percent.

So genetics appears to account for a sizable chunk of the tendency to develop social phobia, but leaves at least half of the influence to various environmental factors. A variety of environmental factors could potentially influence the development of social phobia. These include exposure of the fetus to viruses, drugs, or nutrients that might affect brain development, and later exposure to a particular upbringing by parents, observing and learning from the social behaviors of parents and classmates, and any traumatic experience of humiliation.

It is also important to recognize that these estimates of genetic versus environmental influences only describe statistical averages for the population as a whole. If genes control 30 percent of the overall chance of getting social phobia, for any one person with social phobia, genes theoretically could account for very little or very much of that one person's tendency toward social anxiety. We say "theoretically" because such calculations are not currently possible in regard to individuals. In some persons social phobia may be largely inherited, and in others it may be largely learned.

SOCIAL PHOBIC BABIES?
THE INHIBITED TEMPERAMENT

Another way to separate inherited factors from environmental ones is to study babies before the environment has had a chance to make a full impact. The study of shy children at the Harvard Infant Study Laboratory has provided additional evidence for a genetic contribution to social anxiety.

In the 1960s, child psychologist Jerome Kagan noticed that observations of children as they developed from birth to adolescence had shown only one psychological quality that was preserved from the first three years of life through adulthood—a shy temperament. "Temperament" refers to the inborn, characteristic way in which an infant responds to its environment, the infant's budding personality style. Kagan observed in a study of day care in China that Chinese infants were more subdued, shy, and fearful than Caucasian infants when encountering unfamiliar people, and they also had more elevated heart rates—one of the features of shy temperament. He decided to focus on this phenomenon, which he called "behavioral inhibition," in greater detail in the 1980s. The results have proven intriguing.

From a group of children as young as twenty-one months old, Kagan selected out two subgroups on the basis of tests of their temperament—the toddler version of personality testing. Children who were consistently shy, quiet, and timid when they were exposed to unfamiliar people and objects were considered to have a behaviorally inhibited temperament. Those who were consistently sociable, talkative, and emotionally spontaneous in the same setting formed the opposite, a behaviorally uninhibited group. The 15 percent of the children who were at each extreme of this spectrum were selected for further study.

The inhibited temperament proved to be fairly stable over time. When these children were tested again at age seven, 77 percent of the behaviorally inhibited kids remained more quiet, serious, cautious, and shy than average. Of the kids who were inhibited at both age two and age seven, two thirds remained inhibited on repeat testing at age twelve to fourteen. It was uncommon for an inhibited toddler to cross over to the other extreme of sociability.

Kagan theorized that these stable behavioral differences in such children reflected inborn differences in brain function. He suggested that areas of the brain that were known to cause fear reactions, such as the amygdala, might be activated more easily in the behaviorally inhibited children. High activity in these areas of the brain would lead to activation of the sympathetic nervous system, the part of the nervous system responsible for the release of adrenaline into the circulation and the resulting fight-or-flight response.

If Kagan's theory was true, increased sympathetic nervous system activity would be detectable in inhibited children by specific physiological measurements. As predicted, the children showed higher heart rates at rest, more heart rate acceleration and greater increase in pupil size in response to unfamiliar people and objects, and higher levels of breakdown products of the neurotransmitter noradrenaline in their urine. The inhibited children also had higher levels of a circulating hormone, cortisol, that is typically released in response to stress and that was measured in the children's saliva.

Skeptics said this data was very interesting, but it didn't prove that these biological differences had been present from birth. Perhaps differences in early rearing by parents could have already caused such inhibited behavior. Kagan's group went back to the lab to study the responses of four-month-old infants to a variety of novel stimuli. About 20 percent of these infants showed a pattern of high reactivity to stimulation, with vigorous movement and fretting or crying. When they were retested at age three, these high-reactive infants were more likely to be shy and inhibited. Finally, Kagan reported that his group had gone all the way back to the womb and found that fetuses with higher heart rates three weeks before birth are also more likely to become inhibited babies.

This inhibited temperament appears to be a risk factor for the development of social phobia and other emotional problems in older children and adults. Inhibited toddlers followed up three years later had more anxiety disorders, including social phobia. In a study of the families of Kagan's children, parents of the behaviorally inhibited children had a rate of social phobia (18 percent) that was significantly higher than the rate among a control group of parents of children in the community (3 percent). Some other emotional problems, such as panic attacks, were also more common.

These findings on behavioral inhibition have important implications for our biological and psychological understanding of social anxiety and social phobia. From a biological perspective, inhibition may offer a window into the genetic and physiological factors that underlie social anxiety before they become obscured by years of environmental influences. So further study of behavioral inhibition may begin to reveal the specific genetic and other biological factors that underlie shy behavior. Uncovering the brain and body chemistry that lead to behavioral inhibition holds the potential for development of more effective treatments that target the biological root causes of social phobia.

From a psychological perspective, behavioral inhibition could be equally important, but for different reasons. If a toddler with behavioral inhibition is at risk for developing social anxiety problems later in life, early identification could help parents adapt their approach to the child in order to head off future problems. Parents might be educated in child-rearing techniques that have been shown to counteract a child's tendency toward social fear and avoidance. These include avoiding overprotection and encouraging such children to enter unfamiliar situations while helping them develop coping skills. It is commonly accepted that parents can make their normal children neurotic, so shouldn't they be able to help "neurotic" infants grow up better adjusted? We will discuss advice for parents of shy children in chapter 17.

IS THERE A UNIQUE PHYSIOLOGY OF SOCIAL ANXIETY?

Regardless of the underlying genetic or environment causes of social anxiety, an adult's actual experience of social anxiety usually includes physical symptoms. As we have discussed, symptoms such as blushing, a racing heart, tremors, and sweating are caused by hormonal and nervous system activation. But is this physiology unique to social anxiety, or are we just feeling generally activated but label this activation "social anxiety" because of the social circumstances in which it occurs? The pendulum of scientific opinion has swung between these explanations over the past century.

Toward the end of the nineteenth century, the American psychologist William James and the Danish physiologist Carl Lange independently arrived at an idea that has come to be known as the James-Lange theory. As James put it, "Common sense says, we lost our fortune, are sorry and weep; we meet a bear, are frightened and run; we are insulted by a rival, are angry and strike. . . . My theory . . . is that the bodily changes follow directly the perception of the existing fact, and that our feeling of the same changes as they occur *is* the emotion . . . we feel sorry because we cry, angry because we strike, afraid because we tremble. . . ." According to this theory, an embarrassing event would lead directly to bodily changes such as blushing and trembling, and we would feel embarrassment as we became aware of these specific symptoms.

By the early 1960s, the pendulum was swinging in the other direction. Psychologists Stanley Schachter and Jerome Singer devised an experiment in which two groups of volunteer subjects were given a stimulant drug. Within each group of subjects, one person was actually a confederate of the experimenter. In one of the groups, after taking the drug the confederate performed some wild antics to suggest to the subjects that he was in a state of euphoria. In the other group, the confederate expressed anger in front of the other subjects, tearing up a form and stomping out of the room. The results of the study showed that unknowing subjects were more likely to report experiencing whichever emotion they had seen the confederate display. The experimenters concluded that it wasn't the particular physiological effect of the stimulant drug that determined the emotional experience, but that labeling the emotion depended instead mainly on the social surroundings.

In regard to anxiety, it once was widely believed that a single physiological state of stimulation was the basis for all forms of fear or anxiety, such as fear of being attacked, fear of the sight of blood, fear of suffocating in a crowded elevator, or fear of embarrassment while giving a speech. More sophisticated recent studies have demonstrated, however, that different physiological states accompany different kinds of anxiety. It turns out that all anxiety is not alike.

For example, people with panic disorder suffer spontaneous bursts of anxiety that often share some symptoms with social anxiety—such as a pounding heart, increased heart rate, and tremor. But other symptoms separate the two syndromes. Unlike persons with social phobia, panic disorder sufferers commonly experience difficulty breathing, chest pain, choking, dizziness, and fear of dying or passing out. People with social phobia are more likely to experience other symptoms, such as blushing or twitching muscles, during their anxiety episodes.

Differences between panic disorder and social phobia have also shown up in the laboratory, where chemical probes of the anxiety system have different effects. For example, when certain chemical substances, such as sodium lactate or caffeine, are given intravenously to people with panic disorder, most will have a panic attack within minutes. This is primarily a physiological response, rather than just mind over matter, for when the same subjects are given an inert saltwater placebo intravenously instead of the chemical substances, they are unlikely to experience panic. Persons with social phobia, however, like persons with no anxiety problems, are unlikely to get an anxiety attack from the chemical substances.

So there is growing evidence that specific types of anxiety problems are related to specific patterns of physiological responses. Building on the theories of James and Lange and Schachter and Singer, current research suggests that our emotions are based on specific physiological responses *and* may be modified by the environment in which they are experienced. Easily detected physical symptoms such as blushing and trembling might serve as starting points from which to trace the physiology that underlies the experience of social anxiety.

THE ADRENALINE HYPOTHESIS

Many social anxiety symptoms (increased heart rate, palpitations, tremors, sweating) can be grouped as activation of what is known as the sympathetic nervous system. When this system is activated, it stimulates the adrenal glands to produce the hormone adrenaline, which then circulates throughout the bloodstream. The circulating adrenaline and direct nerve messages from the brain to vital organs are responsible for the symptoms of the fight-or-flight response. Could adrenaline be the essential source of social anxiety?

Blood adrenaline levels have been shown to increase dramatically in most people during performance activities such as public speaking, and medications known as beta-blockers, which block the effects of adrenaline, can stop the symptoms of stage fright from developing. These medications work by attaching themselves to beta-receptors on various organs, such as the heart and sweat glands. They physically block adrenaline molecules from becoming attached, thus preventing the receptors from being activated.

It seemed possible that persons with social phobia might be prone to social anxiety symptoms because they either produced too much adrenaline or were more sensitive to its effects than other people. To test whether adrenaline might cause social anxiety, psychiatrist Laszlo Papp at New York State Psychiatric Institute gave adrenaline intravenously to volunteers with social phobia. As expected, blood adrenaline levels increased greatly, but the subjects did not experience intense symptoms of social anxiety. It seems that the physiological arousal of an adrenaline surge alone is not enough to trigger the symptoms of social anxiety. Perhaps, to have full effect, adrenaline levels need to be increased in the brain itself. Alternatively, along the lines of the earlier work of Schachter and Singer, adrenaline production may contribute to social anxiety only when it occurs in a stressful social situation.

THE ANXIOUS HEART

Another way to study the physiology of social phobia is to measure what is going on in a person's body during the natural experience of social anxiety. Because attaching wires and drawing blood samples from people at cocktail parties would be awkward, messy, and might take the fun out of the party, researchers have attempted to provoke social anxiety in the more convenient setting of their own laboratories. A favorite approach has been to simulate a public speech by asking research subjects to give a talk in the laboratory. In one study, persons with social phobia and control subjects who were free of social anxiety problems volunteered to be tested while giving a ten-minute speech to a small audience of laboratory staff. Blood samples were taken from each speaker at regular intervals through a small intravenous line.

The two groups showed no differences in blood levels of adrenaline or other stress hormones that were measured before and during the speeches.

One unexpected finding, however, which has now been confirmed in studies by several research groups, is that people with different types of social phobia show different patterns of heart rate reactions to public speaking. Persons with performance anxiety experience a surge in heart rate during the first minute of a performance situation. This is less pronounced, however, for persons with the generalized form of social phobia, even though their fear of public speaking is just as severe. So there may be two kinds of people with social phobia, each with different physiological reactions. One group may be particularly prone to surges in physical symptoms, such as a racing heart, blushing, trembling, and sweating, especially in performance situations such as giving a speech. The other group may have less severe physical responses but more worrisome thoughts about how they are being judged in both particular performance situations and social situations in general. It remains to be seen whether the two groups will show different responses to particular treatments.

TRACING THE BLUSH

If any particular symptom holds the key to the physiology of social phobia, blushing might be it. Blushing is one of the most characteristic symptoms of embarrassment, and not surprisingly, some people with social anxiety complain of blushing too much. Blushing also provides more evidence that social fear has a different physiological basis than other kinds of fear. In fear responses to physical danger, people often turn pale because the blood vessels in the face constrict. Just the opposite seems to be true in fears of social criticism or embarrassment.

The actual physiological mechanism of blushing is poorly understood. Blushing is believed to be the result of an increase in the volume of blood in vessels just beneath the skin. This filling of the blood vessels depends on relaxation of the muscle tone in the blood vessel walls. The muscle relaxation is in turn controlled by the vessels themselves and by the influence of adrenaline circulating in the bloodstream. The naturally elastic quality of surface blood vessels in the "blush region" (the face, ears, neck, and upper chest) may explain why blushing is usually localized to this area.

Blushing, of course, is not the only signal of embarrassment. Scientists in the laboratory are learning to describe what any shy child can perform without training—the facial expression of embarrassment. A full display includes averting one's gaze, shifting the eyes rapidly, touching the face, covering the mouth, and showing a nervous, silly smile that reaches its peak after the gaze is averted. Despite the smile, research studies have shown that observers can distinguish facial expressions of embarrassment from expressions of amusement. Embarrassed subjects look down more than amused subjects, shift their gaze more frequently, show efforts to control or turn off their smiles, and turn their heads away or down more. Observers watching videotaped facial displays can reliably distinguish embarrassment from a variety of other emotions, including amusement, shame, anger, disgust, and enjoyment. It remains to be seen whether facial displays of embarrassment are consistent across different cultures, as has been shown for some other basic emotions.

IS DOPAMINE THE SHYNESS CHEMICAL IN THE BRAIN?

Another approach to uncovering the biological underpinnings of social phobia is to search for chemical factors that trigger the social anxiety signal at its origin in the brain. Most of the medicines that are helpful in the treatment of social phobia appear to work via their effect on neurotransmitters, the natural chemical messengers that carry signals from one nerve cell to another within the brain. Nardil and other MAO (monoamine oxidase) inhibitor medications prevent the deactivation of certain neurotransmitters—such as dopamine, norepinephrine, and serotonin—thereby increasing their effects. Klonopin and other benzodiazepine medications interact with the target of the neurotransmitter GABA (gamma aminobutyric acid) to quiet anxiety pathways in the brain. Prozac and related drugs work by blocking the retrieval of the neurotransmitter serotonin from the space between nerve cells into nerve cells, which results in increased effects of serotonin. Although these medicines work in different ways, they all have the end result of "turning the volume down" on the social anxiety signal. It is possible that these drugs work in social phobia by correcting a preexisting deficiency or excess of a particular neurotransmitter in the brain, but the specifics of such an abnormality have been elusive.

One hypothesis proposed by psychiatrist Michael Liebowitz is that dopamine is the neurotransmitter culprit in social phobia. In depressed patients, levels of dopamine in the spinal fluid, which bathes the brain and spinal cord, were found to be lower in those patients who were less extroverted. This suggested that the low extroversion of social phobia sufferers might relate to their lower levels of brain dopamine. Another study questioned patients with Parkinson's disease, whose tremors are known to be caused by a deficiency of dopamine in one specific region of the brain, about any previous problems with anxiety. Seventeen percent of these patients reported having had significant symptoms of social phobia before the start of Parkinson's disease, a higher rate than expected. This suggests the possibility that an early, subtle deficiency in the dopamine system might have predisposed these patients to the development of social phobia well before the deficiency progressed into the more extreme range and resulted in Parkinson's disease. It is not known, however, whether people with social phobia get Parkinson's disease more often than would otherwise be expected.

In an animal model of social phobia, a strain of mice was bred for low aggression over more than twenty-five generations. These mice would become inhibited and freeze in response to mild social contact with an unfamiliar mouse. (While humans tend to think of all mice as mousey, mice apparently think this is relative.) The brains of these "shy" mice differed from the brains of normal mice primarily in having lower levels of the neurotransmitter dopamine.

Dopamine in the brain is important for motivating pleasure-seeking activities and the curiosity to enter unfamiliar situations. This has been shown in laboratory studies testing animals' motivation to work for rewards, such as by pressing a bar to obtain food. Animals low in brain dopamine are less willing to work hard for a reward, and they are also less interested in exploring novel features in their environment, like a new toy. Liebowitz has theorized that low dopamine might similarly interfere with the social motivation of persons with social phobia. While people with social phobia desire relationships, they seem less able to see past the risk of approaching a stranger to the potential rewards of social interaction. The dopamine theory of social phobia is supported by the effectiveness of MAO inhibitor medications, which increase brain dopamine activity. But although it is intriguing, the theory needs more testing before we can conclusively link the dopamine deficiency of rodents to the social phobias of people.

Dopamine is not the only biochemical candidate for a leading role in social phobia. Other studies have suggested that the neurotransmitter serotonin is important in this area. In animals, serotonin has been shown to be crucial to the brain chemistry that underlies social dominance hierarchies, the pecking orders within social groups that seem analogous to some human social strata. As we discussed in chapter 8, social anxiety may have originally evolved in monkeys as an adaptive response that protected lower-ranking individuals from attack by dominant members of a hierarchy.

THE CHEMISTRY OF DOMINANCE

Researchers Michael McGuire and Michael Raleigh have conducted a series of studies examining the interaction of brain chemistry with social behaviors in a captive colony of vervet monkeys. In stable social groups of vervet monkeys, individuals with higher levels of brain serotonin tend to engage in more mutual grooming and other friendly social activities. Treatment of these monkeys with Prozac (or with other drugs that tend to increase serotonin activity) increases the frequency of the same friendly social activities.

Vervet monkeys naturally form dominance hierarchies in which rank has its privileges. In these hierarchies, the higher-ranking animals are often accorded their choice of food, sleeping sites, and social partners. When a reigning dominant male dies or loses influence (every eighteen months, on the average, for this species in the wild), a competition ensues to determine which male will take his place.

Raleigh studied the effect of serotonin on the competition for dominance by removing the dominant males from twelve social groups, each of which had originally included three males. He then tested the effects of two different drugs on one of the two remaining males in each group. Each drug was given for four weeks, with time in between for the effects of the first drug to wear off. One drug increased serotonin activity; the other drug decreased it. During every four-week period when an animal received the serotonin-increasing drug, it became dominant over the other (untreated) male of the pair. During every four-week period when an animal received the serotonin-decreasing drug, it became subordinate to the other (untreated) male.

How did the drugs influence the monkeys' social fortunes? Raleigh noted that the treated monkeys tended to follow the same three steps to achieving dominance that occur naturally in the wild: First they increased friendly social interactions with females, then they obtained increased support from females during conflicts with other group members, and finally they defeated the other male in physical battle.

Serotonin levels may be much less important in determining changes in dominance status in stable social groups, where there is no vacancy for the top position. This was shown in another study, in which low-ranking monkeys in a stable social group were treated with drugs that increased their serotonin. After treatment, these low-ranking monkeys were ostracized less by the group, and they engaged in more friendly behavior than before. However, while they sometimes rose in rank, they did not become dominant.

But do these studies mean anything for people? It is useful, of course, to remember that we differ from monkeys. Social and cultural factors—such as upbringing, privilege, education, traditions, and prejudice—greatly affect who wields power over whom in human social groups. These factors may override or diminish the impact of pure biology.

No matter how cultured we are, however, we remain cultured animals, and our actions are influenced by our evolutionary heritage and brain chemistry. As we discussed in chapter 8, people with social phobia do share certain characteristics with other social animals dissatisfied with their position in a dominance hierarchy. It seems certain that a piece of the puzzle of human relationships and hierarchies is related to differences in brain chemistry. The most powerful evidence for the influence of brain chemistry is the recently discovered effectiveness of a variety of medications for social phobia, as we will discuss in chapter 19.

MEASURING BRAIN CHEMISTRY INSIDE OUT

In people, neurotransmitters are difficult to study because they cannot readily be measured in the brain itself, but indirect methods to measure them have become increasingly sophisticated. While the brain seems to have been designed with natural protection against dangerous intruders, including neuroscientists, it has been possible to test spinal fluid and blood to measure changes in levels of by-products of the breakdown of neurotransmitters. These by-products may reflect activity of the responsible neurotransmitter in the brain.

Measurement of neurotransmitter breakdown products in people with other psychiatric conditions, including depression, panic disorder, and obsessive-compulsive disorder, has sometimes demonstrated abnormal regulation of these neurotransmitters. Some of the few studies so far conducted in persons with social phobia have suggested an abnormality in the serotonin system. The studies have not firmly established any abnormality as unique to social phobia, however, and much work remains to be done. Additionally, the significance of these indirect measures of neurotransmitters, such as measures of their breakdown products in the blood, is often uncertain. Critics have likened this approach to trying to understand the political policy of the White

House by analyzing the contents of one of its garbage cans (including documents that have passed through the customary paper shredder).

Instead of just taking a "snapshot" by measuring neurotransmitter levels at a single point in time, a more dynamic approach tests the functioning of a neurotransmitter system by challenging it with a single dose of a particular drug. The neurotransmitter system reacts to the drug by releasing certain hormones into the bloodstream. Based on the resulting changes in levels of specific hormones in the blood, the activity of the brain neurotransmitter system that accounts for that response can be estimated.

Even these techniques have serious limitations. Because neurotransmitters all carry on important interactions with one another, a primary abnormality in the level of one neurotransmitter might secondarily show up in levels of other neurotransmitters and other chemical substances in the brain. Many active neurotransmitters probably remain to be discovered and cannot yet be measured. Finally there is location, location, location. The activity level over the brain as a whole (as reflected in the spinal fluid) may be normal for a particular neurotransmitter system, yet this may belie variations within regions of the brain that could be causing significant problems.

PICTURING SOCIAL ANXIETY IN THE BRAIN

There is a new way of looking inside the brain that circumvents some of these pitfalls: brain imaging. The latest methods include positron emission tomography (PET), single proton emission computerized tomography (SPECT), and magnetic resonance imaging (MRI). These techniques allow more precise measurement of brain structure—and in some instances even brain chemistry.

Psychiatrists at Duke University recently used MRI to study various brain regions in patients with social phobia. One small structure that is known to be involved in the emotion circuitry of the brain, the putamen, was found to decrease in size with age in patients to a greater extent than in normal control subjects. The putamen, normally about half the size of a Brazil nut, is made up of a group of cells deep in the brain. It includes many dopamine-containing nerve cells, so a smaller-sized putamen in social phobia would go along with the hypothesis that low dopamine is related to this problem.

These are intriguing findings, and brain-imaging technology could ultimately lead to a much better understanding of the physical underpinnings of social phobia. But these findings are also very preliminary, and there are still pitfalls in the interpretation of complex computer-generated scans. Thus, these first results need to be replicated before we can draw any firm conclusions.

What is clear at this point is that social anxiety and social phobia are biological as well as psychological and social phenomena. They have a genetic component, and we have uncovered some tantalizing clues to their physiology and brain chemistry. At present, however, these clues do not clearly point to a useful diagnostic test or help us choose a treatment for any individual patient. They do hold the potential, however, for leading us to more specific and more effective medication and psychotherapy treatments for social phobia. For example, it might turn out that there are several different types of brain chemistry that can predispose a person to what we now generically call social phobia, but each type might respond best to a particular medication, or perhaps even to a particular psychotherapy approach. With new diagnostic tools, it might become possible to eliminate any guesswork and to direct a person immediately to the specific treatment that is most likely to succeed.

PSYCHOLOGY OF THE SHY

We are what we repeatedly do. Excellence, then, is not an act, but a habit.

Aristotle

In this chapter we examine the social anxiety beast from several different psychological perspectives. One test of any psychological theory is how well it can explain a person's actual social behavior. Does the model fit with your own experience? Does it predict what you would do in certain situations? Can it possibly help you manage your social fears?

Every infant enters the world with a particular inborn temperament, but that world immediately begins to influence social development through the baby's first interactions with its parents. Soon, the child also learns to imitate social behavior by watching how parents and siblings mix with others. Throughout the life span, stressful life events—from a school yard humiliation to the death of a loved one to a job promotion—may dramatically reshape a person's social possibilities and demands. All of these influences lead to the development of social attitudes and behaviors—our typical ways of thinking and doing—which in turn affect the outcome of our subsequent social encounters. Discovering how such psychological factors relate to social fears can help change troubling behaviors and thinking patterns.

The same type of understanding has led to therapies to overcome social phobia.

YOU ARE WHAT YOU DO: THE RULES OF BEHAVIOR

One approach to understanding social anxiety begins with study of the simpler concerns of rodents and monkeys. Behavioral psychology explains the impossibly complex development of human social anxiety by breaking anxiety down into discrete behaviors. Behavioral models, which try to predict such behaviors, have the advantage of lending themselves to scientific testing. These models put aside the black box of human consciousness (and we will put it aside temporarily) and start with the premise that what people *do* is the key to understanding their problems. This behavioral approach forms the foundation for cognitive-behavioral models that recently have gained prominence in explaining and treating social phobia.

Not long after the famous Russian behaviorist Ivan Pavlov trained dogs to salivate to the sounds of a metronome by pairing the sounds with the presentation of meat, others began to apply his method of learning by association to study fears. The case of Little Albert is a famous early behavioral experiment on development of fear, although its methods are abhorrent by today's ethical standards for research. Albert was eleven months old and living in an orphanage at the time of this study in the 1920s. J. B. Watson, a founding father of behavioral psychology, rang a loud bell while simultaneously placing a furry white rat in front of Albert's eyes. While the bell had previously frightened the child, the rat had not. After the bell and the rat were paired, however, Albert developed a persistent fear, not only of rats, but also of white furry objects in general, including cats, dogs, and even a handful of wool.

This way of picking up a fear is known as **classical conditioning,** and it can explain a wide range of fears. A cancer patient who visits a hospital for chemotherapy treatments that cause nausea and vomiting may be surprised to discover that nausea and vomiting later occur whenever he walks past any hospital. In this instance, an emotionally charged experience (chemotherapy-induced vomiting) and a previously neutral situation (being near a hospital) have become powerfully linked in the person's mind.

The same pairing can occur with social fears. Mark was a graduate student who had outgrown childhood shyness to become outgoing and personable. He had always been confident in interviews, but one day he felt jittery and stammered during an important job interview. The interviewer, instead of being sympathetic, was sadistic. He told Mark that he was obviously immature and troubled, and that he had no business interviewing for such a prestigious and demanding job. Following this painful humiliation, Mark discovered that just the thought of an upcoming interview, no matter what the pressure level, produced an automatic response of panic.

Once they are paired with a particular situation, intense fears can be incredibly persistent, even when the pairing is irrational. Social fears in particular seem easy to acquire but difficult to shed, perhaps for reasons deep in our evolutionary history, as we discussed in chapter 8. For Mark, the unexpected harshness of the criticism he received was especially traumatic, forging a strong link for him between being interviewed and feelings of extreme anxiety. Fortunately for Mark, he was able to work on pairing new positive emotional experiences with interviews, and eventually he made good progress. Little Albert, on the other hand, left the orphanage shortly after Watson's experiment, and the world may never know whether he ultimately overcame his phobia of white fur.

We do know from several research studies that about half of all people with social phobia recall a traumatic event that seemed to set off their problem. These traumatic events usually involve an experience of humiliation in a social situation, such as being laughed at by the entire second grade class after losing bladder control during a show-and-tell presentation. Adults with a specific social fear, such as fear of public speaking, appear more likely to recall a traumatic event than adults with generalized social fears. It is not possible to draw firm conclusions about the origins of social anxiety from these studies, however, because of the unreliability of early childhood memories and because embarrassing experiences may be more traumatic for children who are already shy.

REWARD AND PUNISHMENT: THE TWIN MOTIVATORS

In many people with social fears, no such traumatic trigger can be identified. Instead, the fears seem to have crept into a person's life gradually. A variation of the classical conditioning theory, **operant conditioning,** explains these fears as the culmination of a long series of small negative experiences rather than a response to a single traumatic event.

Beginning in the late 1920s and early 1930s, psychologist B. F. Skinner was refining the principles of operant conditioning at Harvard by teaching pigeons to play Ping-Pong and rats to do just about anything. His type of conditioning, really a form of learning, involves the use of rewards to encourage a particular behavior. Skinner believed that all behaviors, including fearful responses, have been shaped in predictable ways by past experience of the *consequences* that followed the same behaviors. If a rat receives an electric shock (a punishment) when it visits one part of a cage, it will avoid that part of the cage in the future. If the rat receives a food pellet (a reward) when it visits another part of a cage, it will visit there again.

People respond to operant conditioning as well. If we have grown up receiving praise and rewards from our parents, teachers, and friends for particular social behaviors, such as giving public presentations, we are more likely to be comfortable speaking up in front of others. If we have received frequent criticism (a punishing consequence) for the way we talk, we are more likely to develop fear and to shy away from formal speaking.

While the notion that our previous experience of rewards and punishments influences the likelihood of our current social behaviors may seem obvious, this idea often runs counter to how most people think. People tend to identify a feeling or an event that occurred *just prior* to a particular behavior as its critical "cause." Harry would say "I cut my speech short because I was nervous," rather than "I cut my speech short because I have a history of experiencing relief of anxiety when I stop speaking." In the latter view, it is the reward of relief that influences Harry's behavior.

So what's the point of these fine distinctions? While classical conditioning models ask the socially anxious person to recall early traumatic events that triggered social fear and avoidance, the operant model asks what may seem quite strange at first: "What consequences, positive or negative, do I experience by entering and leaving social situations?" Although the consequences Harry thought about the most were feeling humiliated and putting himself down for failing at his speech, the little-noticed consequence of short-term relief from anxiety was also driving his unwanted behavior. For Harry, relief was spelled E-S-C-A-P-E. Harry's avoidance relieved his unpleasant anxiety symptoms and prevented him from possibly having to endure critical looks or comments from his audience.

Rather than emphasizing the influence of complex emotional experiences like fear and anxiety, classical and operant conditioning models emphasize the influence of specific problem behaviors. A young student whose teacher often criticizes his answers to questions will begin to avoid raising his hand in class. A girl whose singing is repeatedly ignored or mocked in elementary school is less likely to feel confident about her ability to participate years later in the high school choir. She may even grow to avoid other activities that involve singing, such as joining friends to go Christmas caroling.

The same conditioning models provide a basis for methods to change unwanted behavior. So, for example, the often criticized child might become more eager to raise his hand if his teacher were to praise the parts of his answers that are acceptable; the little girl who liked to sing might cope better if others responded more positively to her attempts. By focusing on specific behavior, these models skirt the inscrutable complexity of the internal workings of the mind and brain.

The simplicity of behavioral models, while elegant, has been challenged by those who believe that in order to understand people, thoughts and feelings need more attention. "Cognitivists" point out that all the praise in the world won't erase a social fear if the fearful person rejects the praise and clings to irrational fears of embarrassment. Moving inside the "thinking mind" of anxiety provides different ways to explain and manage social fears.

YOU ARE WHAT YOU THINK: THE COGNITIVE CONNECTION

Moments before Harry enters the banquet room where he is to make a toast, several unwanted negative thoughts invade his consciousness: "What if I forget what I had planned to say? They will think I am a fool. . . ." Harry begins to tremble, and he is convinced that others will notice and think he is a nervous wreck. He scans the room to see if his audience had recognized his problem.

When we consider how our thoughts influence what we feel, we are using a **cognitive** model. This model suggests that a tendency to dwell on negative thoughts, which are often inaccurate or untrue, is a cause of negative emotional responses. So, when Harry joins family and friends to make a toast and finds himself thinking "I have nothing impressive to say," his emotions change quickly from a state of confidence to fear, helplessness, and eventually depression.

For some people, these negative thoughts may be part of a pervasive pessimistic view of how they do in social situations. A person with such a negative "cognitive style" might think "Social events always make me nervous" or "I can never think of anything to say when

I'm asked to make a toast." For others, negative thoughts about social situations occur only sporadically and often unexpectedly. Even skilled public speakers who ordinarily enjoy the spotlight may have negative thoughts before a performance such as "They won't like this speech" or "I could fumble and forget what I was about to say." These thoughts are immediately followed by tension and anxiety, but they typically dissipate after the first minute or two of the speech.

Whether constant or sporadic, fearful thoughts often appear to arise in an automatic fashion, much like the conditioned nausea of the chemotherapy patient walking past a hospital. Harry would say "I saw all those guests in front of me and discovered that same terror of embarrassment parked in my head." For Harry and others, the automatic thought is often set off by a particular trigger situation— here, facing the roomful of people. The negative thought also carries the power of any other punishing consequence, like being jeered by an audience . . . only this time, the punishment comes from within. Even if nothing bad actually happens, a preoccupation with negative ideas can be toxic, producing increased fear of a situation that is not actually dangerous.

So if people with excessive social fears are not simply weak willed, as many people assume, but are instead making actual errors in their thinking, this should be testable experimentally. In fact, the notion that socially fearful people think differently from others in social situations has been supported by several independent studies, such as a recent one by psychologist David Clark's research group at Oxford University. The researchers set out to test whether people with social phobia have a negative bias in the way they judge their own ability to converse about everyday activities. They videotaped brief conversations of three groups of people, including individuals with confirmed social phobia, people who were generally anxious but did not have social phobia, and people who had no anxiety problems. Afterward, subjects judged the quality of their conversations and listed any thoughts—positive, negative, or neutral—they recalled having had during the conversation. Psychologist observers watched the videotapes and independently rated the quality of each subject's conversation.

Persons with social phobia had significantly more negative thoughts about their performance compared to the generally anxious and non-anxious subjects. The social phobia subjects also actually performed somewhat less well, but more importantly, they consistently underestimated the quality of their performances. In other words, even when they hadn't done badly, persons with social phobia believed they had made a poor impression on the other person in the conversation. People who always feel badly about their performance deny themselves the positive reinforcement that naturally follows a good performance. This is one way that social phobia interferes with the normal development of self-confidence.

WHERE THINKING GOES ASTRAY

People with social anxiety report that their particular feared situations trigger a wide variety of self-critical thoughts. A few examples are listed below.

TRIGGER SITUATION	AUTOMATIC THOUGHT
Public speaking	"They will think I am a jerk for getting up onstage." "I won't be able to think of anything worthwhile to say."
Going to parties	"My hands will shake so badly that I won't be able to pick up my drink."
Asking someone out	"If she notices me blushing, she won't want to go out with me." "He will think I'm funny-looking." "She will turn me down."
Asking boss for a raise	"Just because it went okay last time doesn't mean I won't blow it this time."

Often these fearful thoughts build on one another. A very competent dentist feared that his hands might tremble noticeably as he performed procedures. His chain of thoughts quickly multiplied from this original idea to the idea that the word would spread among his patients that he could not handle repairing teeth, to the idea that he would lose all of his patients and eventually his practice in bankruptcy court. After losing his practice, he would lose his home and possessions, and his wife and children would leave him in search of a better husband and father. What started as a fleeting negative thought about one unlikely event became a torrent of increasingly negative thoughts. The whole process took only a few seconds and ended with the dentist experiencing his most catastrophic fears with an accompanying surge of anxious feelings.

So why do people care so much about some social situations but not others? According to self-presentation theorists, such as psychologist Mark Leary, people become socially anxious whenever two specific conditions occur in a situation. First, the person must believe it is important to make a good impression on others. Second, the person must doubt his or her ability to make a successful impression. The law student seeking her first job at a firm would be highly motivated to make a good impression. She may feel, in general, that any interviewer would find her likable. If she believes, however, that in this instance she needs to make an incredible impression (and doubts her ability to do so), she is likely to become anxious.

In addition to the *importance* of social presentations, other qualities of social performance make thoughts about this activity particularly vulnerable to distortion. Thoughts about social performance often emphasize either future events or what others think. We can never truly be sure what others think of us, however, and the future cannot be predicted with certainty. Because it is impossible to test the validity of either of these types of thoughts, it can therefore be difficult to recognize the irrationality of social fears. Fears whose irrationality goes unrecognized cannot be dismissed, so they tend to fester.

Socially fearful people often think inaccurately about the future in three general ways. First, they set unrealistic goals for themselves and assume that any achievement short of their goals will be a failure. Second, they overestimate the likelihood that a failure will occur, treating wild speculations as if they were facts. Third, they exaggerate the severity of the negative consequences of such a failure. For example, Harry believes his speech must go perfectly (unrealistic goal). He does not merely wonder about how his speech will actually go, but instead feels sure that he will give a terrible performance (overestimates chance of failure). He does not merely worry that someone in the audience will be disappointed in him, but instead fears the result will be that everyone will think him a fool (exaggerates severity of negative consequences).

An influential originator of cognitive theory, Albert Ellis, argues that most emotional problems are linked to core categories of negative thoughts or presumptions about the world. He boils down these thinking errors to several types of thoughts, such as "I must be perfect" or "I must be loved by everyone." The problem with holding on to such absolute ideas, of course, is that they are impossible to obtain. The person who always "must" do this, or "must" do that, will certainly fail to achieve his or her goals.

But just as the purely behavioral theory had some holes, so does the purely cognitive theory. If these thoughts are so out of line, why don't they get proven wrong by experience? People normally learn from their mistakes. Why do these mistakes go on and on? In recent years, researchers have addressed these questions by a synthesis of cognitive and behavioral theories and their respective therapies. While combined cognitive and behavioral therapies were originally used to treat for depression, similar techniques have now been developed for social anxiety.

THINKING AND DOING: COGNITIVE-BEHAVIORAL MODELS

Cognitive-behavioral models combine both the thinking and doing aspects of social anxiety. They recognize the influence of thinking patterns on social behavior—irrational fears of public speaking obviously will lead to an avoidance of public speaking. Less obviously, they recognize the influence of behavior patterns on fearful thinking. Avoidance of public speaking prevents phobic persons from having the positive experiences necessary to disprove their worst fears, so it ends up reinforcing the very same fears. A therapy approach that attacks problematic thoughts and behaviors simultaneously can have synergistic benefits.

A colleague related a story of attending her first international conference, at which she was to present a paper (on cognitive aspects of anxiety!). At the cocktail party reception, researchers from around the world were socializing in small clusters of three, four, or five people. Our colleague noticed that she was nervous upon entering the large banquet room. When she asked herself why, she recognized that she was having thoughts that everyone else seemed to know one another, that everyone else was having a good time, and that nobody would be interested in her because she was a stranger.

She realized that it was unlikely that nobody at all would be interested in her, so she joined a small group that was engaged in a lively discussion. Unfortunately, these people actually did seem to ignore her, and she felt rejected and stepped aside to regroup. She reminded herself that she could control only her own behavior, not the responses of others, and that people would be more likely to speak to her if she made an effort to speak to them.

Despite her nervousness, she quickly selected another group of attendees, "jumped in," and tried to join the conversation. She spoke nervously and rapidly at first, but eventually she became relaxed and enjoyed the conversation. She ended up becoming good friends with two members of the group and even published a paper with one of them a year later. Her cognitive self-analysis allowed her to change her behavior, and socializing at conferences was thereby "reinforced" both by the tension relief she experienced as she became engrossed in conversation and by the positive, friendly reactions of the other group members.

Just as positive experiences can build confidence, negative experiences can increase fears. People with social fears often recall uncomfortable or even frightening experiences at certain social events. One patient of ours related how an older brother would constantly criticize her behavior at family gatherings: "Why did you look at him that way?" "Don't you know how to talk to people?" She experienced this criticism as punishment, leading to negative views of herself as well as increased social fear and social avoidance.

THE COGNITIVE-BEHAVIORAL HISTORY PERSPECTIVE

According to a cognitive-behavioral history perspective, a person's thoughts and behaviors in any social situation are the products of all that person's positive and negative experiences in similar social situations. An extremely upsetting experience, like tripping and falling into the punch bowl at a party (and viewing it as a humiliating catastrophe), may tip the scale and shift a person from approaching to avoiding similar parties (or punch bowls).

Leon was a sociable sixth-grader who suddenly began avoiding social activities and dances following an embarrassing incident. A known bully had pulled Leon's pants down in the middle of a group of his peers at a local teen center. Leon was mortified, and despite previous positive experiences at school dances, he would blush and become anxious whenever he walked by or even thought about the teen center.

In trying to understand Leon's experience, the cognitive-behavioral view considers Leon's history of positive and negative social experiences, his current way of thinking about the event, and the potential consequences of his avoidance behavior. These three ingredients—*history of consequences* (rewards and punishments experienced from childhood to adulthood), *cognitive style* (characteristic ways of thinking), and *real-life consequences* (rewards and punishments for current behaviors)—all mix like a simmering pot of stew: The individual factors are identifiable, but their effects blend in ways that produce a whole response or feeling.

Leon appeared to develop social phobia as a result of a single traumatic event. But is this really so? In fact, Leon was primed to develop a phobia by some past experiences and a negative cognitive style.

Due to a congenital growth problem, Leon had remained several inches shorter than his peers at school. He was raised by his mother, who worried so much about her son's short stature that she tried to stay by his side always, ready to protect him from the bullies who teased him. As a result of observing his mother's worries about danger, and because his own experience was that his peers were hurtful and aggressive, Leon developed a characteristic way of thinking about other children. He assumed that kids his age would have it out for him. Leon coped by projecting a tough guy image: Anybody who messed with him would pay the price of a fight. His strategy gave him a veneer of self-confidence and respect, but his lack of basic trust made it difficult to find friends.

It was these ways of thinking and behaving (cognitive and behavioral patterns) that Leon carried with him to the teen center dance on that fateful day. While Leon had actually had some good social experiences at two prior dances, during which he'd told a few jokes that were appreciated by his peers, the bulk of his history was that of a child who saw other children as dangerous. It was this child who was suddenly humiliated by a few boys who laughed when another boy pulled down Leon's pants in front of dozens of schoolmates. While Leon had expected the dance to be enjoyable, instead it left him shattered. The reinforcing food pellet (remember Skinner's rats?) became a painful shock instead, and the very sight of the teen center came to elicit devastating memories and unrealistic fears that everybody thought he was a failure.

SOCIAL SKILLS

Sometimes, of course, people with severe social or performance fears are absolutely right when they expect rejection or think they don't know what they are doing: They *do* lack important social skills. Why some people seem to have a harder time picking up particular skills—such as speaking in public, asking someone for a date, or performing onstage—is often unclear, but avoidance can be one factor. People who avoid the situations they fear can fall behind their peers in developing skills because they don't get a chance to practice and learn. People with poor social skills are more likely to both fear embarrassment and get embarrassed.

So although lack of social skills can be a contributing factor, the notion that it is the major cause of social anxiety is not supported by the legions of incredibly skilled individuals who have suffered with social phobias. Few would question Laurence Olivier's ability to act, Barbra Streisand's ability to sing, or former New York Met catcher Mickey Sasser's ability to throw the ball, yet they all publicly disclosed problems with the type of social fear commonly known as stage fright. Besides these anecdotal stories, studies have shown that socially anxious people tend to interpret their social behavior in a negative light independent of its actual quality.

It appears far more common for awkward social behavior to be due to the distraction and interference caused by anxiety rather than to a lack of social skills. Once the anxiety takes over, people forget what they wanted to say and how they wanted to behave. Socially anxious people may come to assume they are simply socially inept, when in reality their fears are inhibiting their otherwise serviceable social skills.

THE THREE-SYSTEM MODEL

While cognitive-behavioral models have the advantage of both looking into the mind and observing behavior, they historically did not directly examine the additional factor of sensations we experience in our bodies. The **three-system model** proposed by psychologist Peter Lang provides an important link between thinking, doing, and physical sensations. Cognitive, behavioral, and physiological factors all combine to create that overwhelming emotion we call anxiety. These factors can operate in different combinations and in different directions.

For the stockbroker who became fearful of making cold calls to potential customers, anxiety could snowball in several ways:

"I'm not up for making calls today." → Palms being to sweat→
   (cognition)   (physiological response)

"I'm sweating, I must be a mess." → Paces around desk →
   (cognition)   (behavioral response)

"They'll notice how nervous I am and think I'm a jerk." →
   (cognition)

Heart pounds, tingling sensations, feelings of unreality →
   (physiological response)

"I'm a mess, I'd better get out of here!" →
   (cognition)

Leaves office → Experiences tension relief
   (behavioral response)   (physiological response)

Some people who are prone to miscalculating the risk of social catastrophes may also tend to be more aware of bodily sensations such as their own rapid heartbeat. Additionally, they may overestimate the likelihood that others will notice a symptom such as blushing or sweating and overestimate the likelihood that others will react negatively if they do notice the symptom. When a disturbing physical symptom, such as blushing, gets relieved by avoidance behavior, such as cutting short a conversation, the symptom relief may act as a powerful reward that encourages future avoidance.

By breaking down anxiety into its component parts, the three-system model is useful for designing programs for change. It is far easier to direct treatments to these particular components than to an amorphous overall experience of anxiety. So we can use cognitive techniques to correct negative ways of thinking, exposure therapy to deal with avoidance, and specific relaxation techniques or sometimes medication to calm physiological symptoms.

The thinking, feeling, and doing model both helps explain why we are feeling anxious at any particular moment and provides a guide for treatment. How do my negative thoughts contribute to my anxiety? What is happening to me physically? What do I do in these feared social situations? This model alone, however, does not explain where these thoughts, feelings, and behaviors develop. Some of the answers lie in childhood.

CHILDHOOD ROOTS OF SOCIAL ANXIETY

How does social anxiety begin? Most children go through a phase of normal social fears. As a child develops the increasing ability to retrieve memories and begins to expect to see certain familiar adult faces, at around six months of age, fear of strange adults develops. In response to a strange face a child may tense up, then burst into tears. This "stranger anxiety" typically peaks at eight to ten months, then gradually disappears by fifteen months. Fear of unfamiliar children overlaps this phase, but usually begins and ends somewhat later. By the time a child is twenty months old, these fears have usually diminished substantially. For some children, however, they may wane very slowly or not at all, developing into true shyness and possibly social phobia.

There may be two stages in the childhood development of embarrassment or social anxiety. The first stage occurs when the child becomes aware of herself or himself as an object that others may look at—by fifteen to eighteen months of age in some children. This form of social anxiety corresponds to adult embarrassment over simply being the focus of attention. It can happen when entering a room where others are already seated, or when being serenaded with "Happy Birthday" by a group of friends. It is related to simply being seen, rather than to being judged badly or humiliated.

A more sophisticated form of embarrassment begins to emerge later, at around age two or three, when children develop the reasoning ability to begin to apply to themselves the rules and standards that govern social behavior. At this stage, for example, a child who is being prompted to greet her uncle, but has forgotten his name, can recognize that she has failed a social expectation. As a result, she blushes and appears bashful, showing what any adult would recognize as embarrassment, although the three-year-old still lacks the verbal ability to describe her feelings in this way.

Many children seem to have been born shy, to have inherited a shy disposition or temperament, as we discussed in chapter 9. Even when shyness has a strong genetic or physiological component, however, it can still be influenced by childhood experiences. One form of environmental influence that has been much studied is overprotection by parents, which has been shown to contribute to childhood fear and avoidance of social activities.

THE INFLUENCE OF PARENTS

Macy reported having been shy for as long as she could remember. As a child she related better to adults than to children her own age. She was keenly interested in what other children were up to but chose to stay on the periphery. Macy would cling to her parents at church or during visits to other people's homes. While her parents permitted this clinging, they would simultaneously criticize her for not playing with the other children.

Numerous studies have found that adults with social phobia tend to recall that their parents were overprotective, forbidding activities that other children were allowed to do, but at the same time providing more criticism than praise. A long-term study of thirty-nine German families found that mothers who were depressed or who were overprotective of their girls during the first two and a half years were more likely to have shy girls at six years of age. The fact that this study did not find the same effect for boys led the researchers to speculate that boys' shyness may be less related to parenting tactics of their mothers.

But why would overprotective parenting put a child at risk for being socially shy and avoidant? Parents who are hyper-concerned about their children tend to isolate them from other children. They discourage them from playing with groups of children and going to parties, and they may emphasize the social dangers involved in these activities, the very training grounds for developing social skills and friends. Every weekend the overprotected child spends alone at home watching TV or playing video games in his or her room is a lost opportunity to learn how to talk to and get along with people other than family members.

Even the most overprotected child, however, will be exposed to some social activity. Imagine this child heading out for a rare party with other children. If the child has maintained a desire to socialize, he or she may see this party as a do-or-die performance event, a performance for which he or she is inadequately prepared. Anxiety grows, and the chance for disappointment is high.

Highly critical parenting may also lead to social fears. Long-term studies that have followed children from the time they were very young have shown that children who saw their parents as rejecting tended to become sensitive to what others might think and say about them. These children often internalize the critical voices of their parents: "I won't have anything worthwhile to say. They'll think I'm stupid for coming to the party." Persistent criticism may lead to a general concern about being judged or evaluated, the central concern of social phobia.

Loretta is a thirty-year-old mother of two with lifelong social fears, particularly of meeting new people and speaking up at formal meetings or in college classes. Growing up as an only child in a military family, she felt that her parents were quite strict and did not encourage her to get out and make friends with other children. Besides being raised by overprotective and uncompromising parents, Loretta had minimal social contacts. This lack of social activity prevented her from practicing the social survival skills needed to gain confidence.

The critical comments that flowed from her parents became part of her "inner megaphone." They became amplified so that any positive thoughts about her social abilities were blocked. As an adult, she remembered telling herself while she was still a child, "I don't know how to talk nicely to adults. I mumble all the time. I'll never be anybody because I only say stupid things. I guess I am pretty stupid." While the inner megaphone blared these negative thoughts, her nervous system would activate anxious feelings, and her natural response was to run and hide. For Loretta, alcohol eventually became a tool for aiding the escape response. But this method only worked in the short run, and it ultimately caused a downward spiral into alcohol-related problems.

Loretta heard her parents' comments as being only negative, but there are great differences in how people accept criticism. Some adults are thick-skinned; they may understand, at least on some level, that seemingly negative comments may actually be well-intentioned attempts to help. They don't like receiving this kind of feedback, but they don't view it as horrible or catastrophic either. Others seem to have been born with a trait of extreme sensitivity to rejection, and they are less able to rationally come to terms with criticism.

Whatever their personalities, children are particularly vulnerable to damage from criticism or rejection. The shy child thinks "If he doesn't want me to come to his house, he must think I'm no fun, and it must be true," and self-esteem is squashed. The experienced but shy adult, who has had the opportunity to develop self-esteem and recognize his own hypersensitivity, may entertain other possibilities: "My initial thought is that he thinks I'm no fun, but I'm overreacting and there is probably some other explanation."

A limitation of most studies of overcritical parenting is that they rely on adults' recollections of how they were treated in childhood. Even if these memories are accurate, the ultimate conclusions of these studies are only as accurate as a child's *perception* of a parent's behavior. Because socially anxious children are very sensitive to critical remarks, they may overestimate the demands their parents and teachers place on them. A child with social phobia might say "I can tell that my teacher doesn't like me because I'm not smart enough," even if the teacher has been generally positive and encouraging. From childhood onward, social fears interfere in this way with a person's ability to collect and analyze social data. Our fearful toastmaster, Harry, for example, may tend to focus on the one or two people in the crowd who appear bored or disinterested during his speech, ignoring the majority, who show pleasure and interest.

Of course, children who are shy from infancy can frustrate the best-intentioned efforts of their parents to promote social activities. Nonshy parents may not be able to relate to shy children's hesitancy to talk with other children or invite them to play. As a result they may begin to push their children, which often results in frustration, more pushing, and ultimately, harsh, critical words. Shy parents, not wanting their children to suffer the same pain they themselves have suffered, may make similar attempts to push their children socially. More often than not, however, they will try to protect their children from anxiety by providing escape routes or by simply keeping them at home and away from others. In this way, parents who are themselves shy may provide home environments that perpetuate shy behavior, amplifying the influences of heredity and environment.

THE FREUDIAN PERSPECTIVE

Psychodynamic models also look to early life experiences as the source of anxieties, although they have had little to say about social anxiety in particular. Freud described symptoms of social phobia in one of his early patients, Frau Emmy von N., but he chose to focus treatment on other symptoms. Freud proposed that phobias, in general, arise out of traumatic experiences that occur in infancy or early childhood and drive disturbing fears and aggressive or sexual wishes into the unconscious. He suggested that the resulting unconscious conflict over these prohibited wishes can come into awareness in the form of anxiety when certain situations occurring much later stir up the old feelings.

The idea that social anxiety is a manifestation of conflict, conscious or unconscious, is consistent with some of the typical ambivalent behaviors shown by an anxious person entering a feared social situation. For example, when he was about to go to the microphone to give his toast, Harry tended to stop and start quite a bit, beginning to stand up, then sitting down again, playing nervously with his hands, before ultimately going ahead with it. In social interactions, a person with social anxiety may intermittently smile and make eye contact, but then turn his or her gaze away prematurely and look down. Often these are not well-thought-out, conscious decisions.

The recognition of unconscious influences on social fears also suggests one way to understand why some people feel embarrassment even when the social attention they receive is quite neutral. For example, the embarrassment some people experience when being introduced during a meeting or when being serenaded with "Happy Birthday" often seems to have no conscious rationale. It is not clear, however, whether such automatic reactions suggest the presence of underlying conflicts, are due to an inborn sensitivity to scrutiny, or have other causes.

The Swiss psychoanalyst C. G. Jung rejected Freud's emphasis on sex as the motivation behind much human behavior, and he introduced the terms "introversion" and "extraversion" to describe two basic personality types. Jung, who classified himself as an introvert, described introversion as a tendency to focus attention inward and on one's inner response to the world. Although he did not emphasize social anxiety as a problem per se, Jung's description of the introvert has many features that overlap with social phobia:

> In a large gathering he feels lonely and lost. The more crowded it is, the greater becomes his resistance. He is not in the least "with it," and has no love of enthusiastic get-togethers. He is not a good mixer . . . He is apt to appear awkward, often seeming inhibited . . . His better qualities he keeps to himself . . . He . . . has an everlasting fear of making a fool of himself, is usually very touchy and surrounds himself with a barbed wire entanglement so dense and impenetrable that finally he himself would rather do anything than sit behind it . . . His picture of the world lacks rosy hues, as he is over-critical and finds a hair in every soup. Under normal conditions he is pessimistic and worried, because the world and human beings are not in the least good but crush him, so he never feels accepted and taken to their bosom. Yet he himself does not accept the world either, at any rate not outright, for everything has first to be judged by his own critical standards.

Modern psychoanalytic theorists have considered some social anxiety to be a manifestation of narcissism. In the person whose anxiety fits this model, self-esteem is dependent on constant praise from others and on feelings of superiority and fantasies of being envied by others, rather than on a less grandiose but more stable inner sense of self-worth. This jerry-rigged self-esteem is vulnerable to collapse at the first sign of criticism or mediocrity. In fact, many persons with narcissistic difficulties spend most of their lives at the lower levels of the self-esteem roller coaster. Such unstable self-esteem may result from a child's insecure attachment to parents who were extremely critical or whose love was conditional upon the child's meeting the parents' needs. As we describe in the following case, a child may "internalize" the beliefs of a critical parent, becoming self-critical and unconsciously assuming that others will be similarly rejecting.

Cynthia, for example, was an attractive twenty-five-year-old accountant who was doing well except for a puzzling absence of the romantic relationship she much desired. All she knew was that she was terrified by the prospect of being rejected by a man. Through the course of therapy, it became apparent that she had gone through two phases in her relationships with men in her adult life. During the first phase she was fairly indiscriminate about whom she went out with, and she would often end up sleeping with a man on their first date in the mistaken belief that this would keep the man interested in her. After many painful rejections and a troubled relationship with a self-centered man who continuously criticized her, she entered the second phase: For the past two years, sure of ultimate rejection, she had avoided all opportunities to meet men despite continuing to long for Mr. Right.

It gradually became apparent that Cynthia's troubles with men were built on the template of her relationship with her father. He was a handsome and gregarious salesman who regarded Cynthia as his favorite child, although due to his travels he spent little time with her. Cynthia's mother had become chronically ill with severe arthritis shortly after their marriage, and the couple slept in separate beds and showed little affection for each other.

As a child, Cynthia loved her father dearly, and when he was home he gave her the admiration her sickly mother was unable to provide. Her father also did things that made Cynthia uncomfortable. Although he was never overtly sexually abusive, he would hold her longer than she wanted to be held, and as she matured, his compliments about her body and her sexiness confused her. When she enjoyed his company, she began to feel she was betraying her mother, and she felt ashamed. When her father left, she would feel she had driven him away with her discomfort.

As an adult, she continued to view him as a nearly perfect father: loving, fun to be with, and a hardworking provider for the family. Through therapy, however, she developed a more complex view of him as a caring father who also had been deeply troubled and sexually inappropriate with her. She came to see one origin of her low self-esteem in having felt rejected whenever her father left for another long business trip. This old hurt feeling would be accompanied by the belief that the discomfort she had felt when her father was around was due to her own flaws, and that these flaws made her unworthy of his love. She had been torn by the unconscious conflict between the desire to please her father and receive his love and the shame she felt at receiving the sexual attention he would not give her mother.

Her adult romantic relationships had become unconscious attempts to play out a happy resolution to her relationship with her father. A part of her felt that if only she would please her boyfriend completely, if only she were more accepting and less self-conscious, he wouldn't leave her like her father had always done. When this strategy failed, her low self-esteem was confirmed. Ultimately she settled for avoidance of entanglements, which prevented the acute pain of a relationship, but at great cost. As she recognized through therapy that the discomfort she had felt with her father was well-founded, she was able to cast off some of the guilt that had burdened her. Awareness of the roots of her troubles allowed her to develop more satisfying romantic relationships, free of the pull toward her old destructive pattern.

Although Freud and his heirs revolutionized the field of psychology, and although psychoanalytic thinking has stimulated tremendous intellectual ferment, the importance of this thinking to understanding and resolving most social anxiety problems remains uncertain. Elements of psychoanalytic theory seem relevant to understanding some forms of social anxiety in some people, but in general they seem less specifically helpful in treatment than the simpler but more testable hypotheses of cognitive-behavioral schools. Political and economic trends have placed psychoanalytic theory and its time-intensive therapies out of fashion. Still, the appeal of psychoanalytic theory lies in its attempt to explain the irrational side of mental processes at a depth beyond that of other theories.

The variety of theories we have reviewed reflects the complexity of social psychology. There is much we do not know. What we do know is that social behavior has multiple influences. Any particular social experience is simultaneously a result of early interactions with our parents, our history of being reinforced and punished for particular social actions, the opportunities we have had to hone social skills, and the way we think and feel about different social situations. All these factors interact with our genes, passed down to us from preceding generations, in developing our social selves.

THE CULTURAL CONNECTION

If society fits you comfortably enough, you call it freedom.

Robert Frost, 1965

Anxiety related to public speaking, talking to authority figures, social-izing, and the like appears to exist in every culture. When mental health professionals from different countries compare notes on social phobia, they find similarities in the fears of embarrassment, the typical age at which this problem begins, and the ratio of men versus women with social phobia. Trembling, blushing, and sweating are recognized around the world as symptoms of social anxiety, as Charles Darwin noted in the nineteenth century. In his work on human emotions, Darwin inquired into the presence of blushing among all the racial groups he could find, including the Lepchas of Sikkim, the Polyne-sians, the Aymara Indians of Bolivia, and the aborigines of Australia. He concluded that blushing is probably common to all races. Based on these similarities across cultures and all the evidence we have already reviewed for individual differences in social anxiety, one might suppose that culture has little to do with social anxiety.

On the other hand, something as social as fear of embarrassment cannot exist apart from the social milieu we call culture. Even if blushing and trembling do have a strong biological basis, and even if life experiences do affect our vulnerability to social fears, we still express these fears through the prism of culture. The effect of culture is evident here in the United States in a simple paradox: Although women are more likely than men to suffer from social phobia, men with social phobia are more likely to seek treatment.

THE GENDER GAP

Social phobia, like most other disorders of anxiety or depression, is far more common among women than men in the general population in the United States—about twice as common, in fact. The reason for this preponderance of women is not known, but there are a variety of possible explanations. The cause may be biological (hormonal differences could make women more vulnerable to certain problems), psychological (women may be more nurturing, more concerned about relationships, and therefore more fearful of loss of the approval of others), and/or cultural (women may tend to be more stressed by social demands such as those of balancing motherhood and working).

The reasons men with social phobia are more likely than women to seek treatment, however, are at least partly cultural. When it comes to problems with anxiety and depression in general, women are more likely than men to seek treatment. This makes the relatively high rate of men seeking treatment for social phobia all the more surprising. Why should men be more likely than women to seek help for problems with shyness or public speaking anxiety, when their general inclination is to avoid the stigma of seeing a "shrink"? Consider the following case:

The vice president of a leading technology company came for treatment, complaining of difficulty giving presentations at high-level board meetings. A suave, handsome, and effective manager, the VP was driven to become president of the company. He was increasingly concerned that his presentations were "merely competent," whereas he thought he should be able to overwhelm the board of directors with his skills. While he hated the idea of seeing an anxiety specialist, he felt that his career was on the line. In his initial visit, he admitted feeling panicked about a rumor that his company's board was considering an outsider for the top position. Through therapy, he was able to recognize that his extreme notion of "overwhelming" the board was creating unrealistic and destructive self-expectations. He worked diligently on therapy homework tasks in which he set goals to demonstrate more cooperative behaviors, and he made significant progress in both reducing his anxiety and solidifying his position at work.

Now consider the revelation of a woman with social anxiety. Annette Funicello, one of the young stars of *The Mickey Mouse Club* television show in the late 1950s, recalls in her autobiography that despite her image of "teen queen," she worried about her extreme shyness. When she asked Walt Disney, her boss and mentor, if she might see a psychologist, he refused. She had a certain charisma, he told her, that depended partly on her shyness. "Going to see a psychologist would change that," he said. "Why do you want to change that?" She never sought treatment.

Despite movement toward sexual equality, men continue to feel that they are expected to exhibit macho qualities such as being aggressive, speaking up in front of groups, and taking the initiative in romantic relationships. While the qualities may be biologically influenced, most cultures also value these qualities more in men than in women. As a result, men tend to experience deficiencies in these qualities as more damaging and distressing. The willingness of socially phobic men to seek treatment, despite the general reluctance of men to admit emotional problems, reflects the intensity of their suffering with shyness.

Women, on the other hand, may find that society, like Walt Disney, has traditionally accepted and even rewarded women who are reticent and take passive roles. Despite substantial strides toward equality, it remains more acceptable for women to avoid taking the lead in the boardroom, ballroom, and bedroom. As a result of these cultural attitudes, women who are limited by social fears may feel less extreme distress than men who are equally fearful. Some women take refuge in traditional feminine roles, but men are more likely to feel they have no place to hide. These differences may diminish as women continue to enter more positions of authority in the workplace and move toward greater equality in the social arena.

A JAPANESE FACE OF SHYNESS

Social anxiety also differs in the form it takes in certain parts of the world. In the 1920s, a syndrome similar to social phobia, called *taijin kyofusho,* was described in Japan by psychiatrist Shoma Morita. *Kyofu* means "fears," and *taijin* has been translated as "social contacts where the exchange of words and glances takes place between individuals." At a symposium one of us (F.S.) chaired on cross-cultural issues in social phobia, a leading Japanese psychiatrist reported that until the term "social phobia" was officially defined and publicized by the American Psychiatric Association in 1979, many Japanese psychiatrists thought the symptoms of social phobia were unique to Japan.

Like people with social phobia, persons with *taijin kyofusho* fear that they will blush, tremble, or sweat in the presence of others. Other *taijin* fears seem more specific to Japanese or East Asian culture. These include fear of emitting a body odor, fear of one's facial expression becoming stiff, and fear of being unable to avoid gazing too directly at people, thereby offending others or making them feel uncomfortable. Sometimes sufferers become quite certain that they are causing others offense. These experiences seem quite odd to most Westerners with social phobia.

There are always exceptions to cultural generalizations, however, as a patient who walked into one of our offices demonstrated just after we had finished the first draft of this chapter. Dirk was a Jamaican-born engineer who had lived in the United States for a decade. By external appearances, he was thriving in this environment. His work was going well, and he was confident of his skills in engineering and office politics. He appeared dapper and spoke eloquently with a charming accent. He was happily married and had just become a father.

Unfortunately, Dirk was also tortured by a particular fear that he felt sure would limit his professional advancement and that had already devastated his social life. He feared that his sweat emitted a body odor so offensive that it would turn colleagues away and cause friends to gossip and have a good laugh at his expense. Yet there he sat describing his problem on a sultry afternoon, appearing cool as a cucumber and odor-free. The irony was not lost on Dirk. He recognized that his fears of embarrassment were excessive and often irrational, yet they seemed beyond his control.

Although the fears seemed beyond his control, Dirk did have some clues to their origins. As a child, Dirk had learned to please his autocratic father with his school achievements but never got the emotional support he desired the most. He had grown up being always the outsider. At boarding school he was shy and the victim of teasing; in his hometown he was the kid from the rich family whom other kids liked to put down. Still, he always had a few good friends, and his keen intelligence brought rewards in school.

As a teenager his various fears of being ostracized became focused on self-consciousness about his bodily odor, and there they remained years later. He could feel comfortable and free of the odor fears only with his closest friends or his wife. In fact, he often asked his wife to inspect him before he would go to a social gathering. If she found him to be odor-free, he felt slightly more relaxed.

In the presence of colleagues or social acquaintances, however, the odor fears were still on his mind. They distracted him from conversation and led him to make excuses to avoid parties. They were strongest in situations with people he most wanted to impress—at meetings with the president of his company or while trying to make new friends. Of course, fear of the odor tended to make him sweat, which increased the fear. His fears could not even be masked by the pungent aftershave he slapped on before going to work. After an episode of severe embarrassment, he would feel depressed and disgusted with his inability to conquer this ridiculous problem.

Although *taijin* fears are not unique to Japan, it is not surprising that social phobia commonly takes this form in Japanese society. Japanese culture has strong conventions regarding offensive social behavior. For example, the act of looking intently at a person during a conversation is considered extremely rude. A tendency to look downward, however, is often appreciated, and may even be considered elegant. Whereas Americans may be self-conscious about failing to make eye contact, Japanese may be more concerned about making eye contact too directly. Across both cultures, however, the person with social phobia experiences excessive fear of breaking the rules of social conduct.

The Japanese are more likely than Westerners to express their social anxiety complaints in an altruistic fashion, through concern about the effect of their awkward behavior on others. This also reflects some of the social pressures in their society. Japanese tend to value hierarchy, politeness, respect for the feelings of others, and self-denial. So social fears in Japan often take the form of concern about making *others* uncomfortable or embarrassed. But like Westerners with social phobia, these sufferers often fear that their inappropriate behavior could also result in their own humiliation.

FACES AROUND THE WORLD

In Saudi Arabia, social phobia has been reported to be particularly common, representing about 13 percent of the people who go to mental health clinics for help (excluding those who have psychotic illnesses such as schizophrenia). Saudis with social phobia appear to have symptoms similar to Westerners', with prominent heart pounding, trembling, and sweating in social situations. The predominance of men seeking treatment is even more extreme in Saudi Arabia than in the United States: In a clinic where two thirds of all other patients were women, men made up 80 percent of patients with social phobia, consistent with the more traditional, private role of women in Saudi society. Kutaiba Chaleby, the Saudi psychiatrist who reported this study, suggested some reasons why social phobia might be so common in his country:

> Saudi culture is heavily disciplined with rigid moral codes and highly valued customs and rituals. Even small deviations from the rules are unacceptable and individuals who do not conform are quickly outcast. It is important to stress that the rules might apply to minor social rituals, such as the manner of greeting somebody, or how to start a conversation by asking about the health of every member of the family, naming only the males and referring to the females by symbols.... Arab culture attaches a great deal of importance to appearances.... One who has made a bad impression in public is likely to retain a poor reputation permanently even though the impression is subsequently shown to have been a false one.... All these factors combined may make those with unique personality traits, or who suffer with a strong sense of individuality, more susceptible to social phobia....

Cultures also differ in their attitudes about social anxiety itself. Westerners tend to stigmatize shyness as a sign of personal weakness, but other cultures view it less negatively. *Layja* is a concept that has been described in Hindu communities in Indian and Nepal. It includes such behaviors as displaying respect for the social hierarchy by acting shy, modest, or deferential; by covering one's face; by remaining silent; or by lowering one's eyes in the presence of superiors. *Layja* is sometimes associated with blushing, sweating, and altered pulse, and it has been translated as "embarrassment," "shyness," or "modesty."

Although Westerners may pity those with social anxiety, many Southern Asians consider *layja* a supreme virtue, especially for women. Like gratitude, loyalty, or respect, *layja* is considered a highly desirable state that maintains social harmony. To be regarded as full of *layja* promotes self-esteem rather than inferiority. In such a society, to be seen as *lacking layja* may be a cause for embarrassment.

Embarrassment is also experienced a bit differently in different cultures, even within the West. British psychologist Robert Edelmann asked study participants from five European countries (Great Britain, West Germany, Greece, Italy, and Spain) to recall how they felt during a recent embarrassing experience. British subjects reported blushing twice as frequently as did persons from other countries. They also tended to report saying significantly less than usual when embarrassed. Italians, Greeks, and Spaniards were more likely to report that they

laugh when embarrassed, but they were least likely to look down
or away.

ANXIETY ON THE MOVE: IMMIGRANTS

Given these differences in cultural attitudes about social behavior, it
is not surprising that immigrants seem particularly likely to experience
problems with social anxiety. First, if they appear different or speak
with an accent, such "otherness" already subjects them to unusual
scrutiny by others. If they bring different social values or if they are
unfamiliar with local social customs, they are also more likely to
commit the gaffe that will draw more attention and even disapproval
from others. Additionally, language difficulties and cultural differences
in communication style may also lead the immigrant to misinterpret
the reactions of others as critical when they are not.

Fresh out of medical school, Oggi decided to escape her native
Hungary (then a Communist country) and seek new opportunities in
America. Upon arriving in New York City, Oggi immediately felt out
of place. She thought that she looked odd in her plain Eastern European clothes (but could not afford new ones), she had no friends, and
she was uncertain about how to do the simplest of social tasks, like
buying milk and bread at the corner grocery store (run by immigrants
from Korea). For the first few months in New York, Oggi spoke only
when it was absolutely necessary, for fear that others would think less
of her because of her strong Hungarian accent and her unpolished
English. With time, Oggi began to feel accepted by fellow members
of the medical community. Oggi's feelings of acceptance followed her
increased identification with a new cultural subgroup, namely the
world of doctors and nurses. Within a few years, Oggi rose to the
ranks of director of a large clinical service at a major medical center.

Of course, you need not come from a foreign country to fall prey
to a culture gap. Leah was a twenty-year-old dance and music student
who recently had arrived in New York City from her native Hawaii.
The daughter of a Hawaiian mother and a part Hawaiian and part
Norwegian father, Leah had excelled in traditional Hawaiian dance
throughout her childhood and young adulthood. In New York, she
quickly found that expectations for both stage appearance and performance were quite different. In addition to declaring her too overweight
to join a prestigious local dance group, her teachers appeared unimpressed with the style of movement she had been taught in Hawaii.
Her self-confidence eroded, and Leah began to experience overwhelming anxiety whenever she was asked to perform. In fact, Leah's teach-

ers believed she had tremendous potential. They had eagerly recruited her, despite her lack of experience with Western-style dance, with the hope of shaping her into a successful dancer. For Leah, the radical shift in place, combined with her sensitivity to critical remarks that had been intended as constructive, overwhelmed the positive views she previously held about herself as a dancer.

In the state of New Hampshire, auto license plates read "Live Free or Die," and the state's residents overwhelmingly support the spirit of the motto. This proclamation of individuality, however, belies the many pressures to act like a traditional New Englander, as one of us (L.W.) discovered upon moving to New Hampshire a few years ago. As an immigrant from New York (locally known as a "flatlander") who had mastered the assertive style of that city, confronting a store-keeper about shoddy merchandise or telling a waitress to send back undercooked blintzes was no problem. Asking new neighbors in the country about fixing a septic tank or using a chain saw, however, was much more awkward. What is an acceptable "New Hampshire" way to ask the same neighbors to keep their barking Dobermans under control or to remove their unsightly abandoned cars from the edge of their property?

This immigrant's confidence was shaken for two reasons: He felt inferior in his ability to perform culturally foreign activities (like fixing a septic tank), and he was unsure of his adopted community's standards for neighborly behavior. At a minimum he risked losing social status, and at worst he could seriously offend his neighbors. This city guy turned country guy experienced disturbing thoughts that had previously been alien to him: "My neighbors will see that I'm incompetent. People here will think I'm a wimp." The physical sensations of anxiety, such as rising heart rate and sweating, began to creep in when he talked with his neighbors and entertained these worries. As he pushed himself to socialize and got to know the neighbors, he realized that simple respect went a long way toward bridging the small culture gap, and the fears eventually eased.

For people who are already shy or have a vulnerability to social anxiety, a move can be the trigger that sets off social phobia. Children who change schools because their family has moved can experience difficulty, even if they are just moving across town. Being the new kid on the block invites scrutiny, and to some that feels like being a deer caught in the headlights. The new child may worry about what is "cool" or "uncool" or how new classmates will respond to his or her appearance or personality.

When Josh's mother, Rebecca, decided to move to the other side of town, she did not realize that this would shift him to a different school district. A child with multiple learning and behavioral problems, Josh had just recently begun to thrive at the local elementary school. He had become friends with two of his classmates and had developed a positive working relationship with his guidance counselor. The thought of going to a new school brought panic to both mom and son. With two weeks remaining in the summer vacation, Rebecca applied for a variance to have Josh remain in his old school—and was turned down. With the help of the special education staff and the school psychologist at the new school, Josh began a series of visits to check out the new school prior to beginning the school year. Once school began, Josh was assigned to a team of "buddies," fellow students whose job was to hang around with him, teach him the new school's routine, and play with him during recess. This planned accommodation helped to relieve Josh's fear of being ostracized.

You need not have just relocated to feel disadvantaged. Both cultural factors and socioeconomic status can influence social anxiety, as has been shown for performance anxiety over taking tests. Although "exam nerves" may not seem to be a form of social anxiety, it shares the crucial component of fear of being evaluated. When such fear of failure and humiliation leads to problems with extreme worry before tests, avoiding tests, or "freezing" while taking them, it is considered a social phobia.

Several studies have compared measures of test anxiety among students of different cultures and socioeconomic groups. Mexican elementary school students have been shown to have greater test anxiety than North American students. A recent study of elementary school students in Chile and the United States found that in both countries students of low socioeconomic status suffered higher levels of test anxiety than middle- or upper-class students. U.S. students overall experienced less anxiety than the Chilean students. The researchers concluded that several factors could account for these differences, including differences in ways of coping with stress, attitudes toward authority figures, and the importance of tests for advancement along professional career paths. These results are consistent with findings of community surveys showing higher levels of social phobia among groups with lower socioeconomic status.

MODERN LIVING, MODERN ANXIETY

Even within mainstream Western (and particularly American) culture, we suspect that a number of influences may contribute to feelings of social anxiety. Increasing mobility causes people to travel in wider circles than ever before, resulting in more frequent brief encounters and a greater need to make a good first impression. The rules of social encounters, meanwhile, have become more fluid, leaving us without traditional guideposts for our social behavior. And to top it off, just as making a good impression is becoming more important and more difficult, unrealistic pressures to achieve flawless performance in our social interactions are growing.

Once upon a time, people judged their competence in comparison to their neighbors. Perhaps a person wasn't as pretty as the girl next door, didn't speak as well in public as the mayor, or felt less successful than the rich folks in town. The advent of global media, however, with its seamlessly efficient distribution of magazines, movies, and television, has bombarded the collective consciousness with an explosion of perfectionistic ideals and inflated expectations. Hundreds of times a day we can compare our bulges, warts, and outdated wardrobe to the supermodels who peddle goods in the modern marketplace. We can compare our stammering speech to sitcom stars who always have a comeback and to newscasters who never say "Um." The problem is that most of us are unable to even approach the level of these stars' illusory looks and speech, so self-consciousness and feelings of inferiority tend to grow.

In earlier times, more people lived in small communities and had direct contact with relatively few others. Their social world was limited, but their own social roles were clear. When a clear social hierarchy was present in a community, people knew where they stood with others, and this stability could be comforting. There is little pressure to impress people whom you and your family have known for years, if not generations.

In today's developed societies, however, we are disconnected from our neighbors. People relocate more and more frequently. Each day we are likely to deal many times with individuals whom we know only superficially, if at all, so we feel the need to make a good first impression more often. Many of these superficial contacts are both first and last impressions—they are as close as we will ever get to the other person. As more of our relationships tend to be fleeting, as in-depth interviews are condensed into television sound bites, making a good first impression soars in importance. More than ever, we rapidly need to let people know who we are. Having firm social customs governing how we present ourselves might make this task easier, but at the same time the rules of social interaction have become more changeable.

If there is one constant in today's social world, it is change. Old-fashioned social conventions, from chivalry toward women to deference toward bosses, have increasingly fallen in the name of equality. Social conservatives reject these trends—but selectively—and some liberals embrace these trends publicly but apply different standards to their own relationships. Unless one retreats to the confines of a like-minded enclave, severing telephone wires and TV cables, and jamming radio frequencies, the overarching trend continues toward an increase in the diversity of what others consider to be acceptable social behavior. Despite the best efforts of Dear Abby and Miss Manners, we have become less certain of what is expected of us.

Just as others' expectations of how we should behave are increasingly difficult to predict, changes in our own social roles create tensions between the new and the traditional, contributing to social anxiety. For example, women have increasingly achieved positions of leadership and power in the workplace. Change seems less dramatic, however, in the social sphere, where shyness is still associated with femininity and women generally expect a man to initiate such activities as dating. How does the modern woman who rises in the ranks of her business or profession reconcile her social and work worlds? To succeed at work she may need to perform in a bold, aggressive way, giving talks in public or engaging in high-pressure sales negotiations. Should she be demure, soft, and self-sacrificing in her personal life but aggressive, hard-edged, and demanding at work? Can she be both, and if so, at what psychological cost?

The conflict for men is less dramatic but analogous. How do boys, encouraged to be socially outgoing and aggressive, and expected to initiate dating or sexual activity, find balance with new expectations to be sensitive and nurturing? Similarly, how does the corporate executive, who is expected to be a tough decision maker who can fire people when necessary, balance this toughness with pressures to be tuned in to the psychological and interpersonal problems of his subordinates? And how does he behave when he returns home as the single parent of a six-year-old son?

FREEDOM IN UNCERTAINTY?

Postmodern psychologists press the case that we are, in fact, many people simultaneously. A tender father is also a tough boss. An aggressive professional woman is also a supportive spouse. Oneness or certainty, as Mary Catherine Bateson has noted, is the exception in twentieth-century life. If there is no one "truth" and no one way to act, then the possibilities are great. There can be liberation in the idea of accepting diversity and disjointedness in life.

Is there a silver lining, therefore, to all this anxiety over the uncertain postmodern rules of social behavior? Perhaps a socially anxious Saudi, feeling suffocated by the web of rules governing every niche of life, would welcome a little ambiguity, a little leeway for social error. Perhaps our socially anxious village-living ancestor, who might have been stigmatized forever by the trauma of going to school in his nightclothes one day in grammar school, would have delighted in the opportunity to uproot to a city, achieve anonymity, and start all over again. Well, yes and no.

If social rules actually are becoming more relaxed, this is a double-edged sword for persons with social anxiety. Relaxing the rules takes away social guideposts, the rules of social etiquette that we use to reduce our anxiety about being embarrassed. On the other hand, greater public tolerance of our "incorrect" social behavior might compensate for the loss of guideposts. Still, rules we can know for sure, no matter how rigid, may feel safer than relying on the tolerance of others, a quality of which we can never entirely be sure. Additionally, while social rules have certainly become more unpredictable, it is not clear that people have become more tolerant to the same extent in their social judgments.

In fact, it seems that when the rules for achieving social acceptance are ambiguous, people work harder to try to get accepted. According to the work of sociologist Erving Goffman, when traditional status symbols (the family name, an individual's reputation for integrity) are unknown, people tend to overcommunicate their group membership for fear of not being understood or properly identified. This communication often takes on a superficial quality; we may use clothing and hairstyles to make statements about our class status, sexuality, tasks, or even political preferences. Consider how people introduce themselves at a party: "Please to meet you, I'm Tom. I'm an attorney with International Inc." or "Where do you live? I live in the Hampton Estates" or "How ya doin'? Did you see the game on Sunday?" Social status or group membership is quickly communicated.

One result of the weight people give these first impressions is that making a poor superficial presentation becomes potentially more damaging. For example, take Vance, who happens to sweat very easily. Living in New York City, Vance gets beads of perspiration on his forehead while riding the subway, even in winter. Some strangers who notice this wonder if Vance is upset about something or if he just sweats easily, and Vance in turn worries that they are thinking something is seriously wrong with him. If he were living in a small village, everyone would know that Vance tends to sweat, but they would also know his family, his character, and his talents. They wouldn't focus on his sweating, and he would be less likely to worry about it.

But what about those benefits of the anonymity of modern city life? Vance has the advantage of knowing he may never see those people on the subway again. Unlike his ancestral villager, he can get a fresh start tomorrow. This is helpful, however, only if Vance can change—if he can ultimately learn to make a better first impression. If not, all his anonymity accomplishes is to allow him to have the same self-conscious anxieties over and over again with new people. And in this community dominated by first impressions, fewer of the people he meets will have a chance to see past the perspiration and get to know the real Vance.

The cultural milieu seems to affect a person's chances of developing social anxiety problems, the way embarrassment is experienced and expressed, and the impact of social anxiety on a person's life. People who differ from the cultural norms in some way—race, clothing, customs, or language—may be at greater risk to develop social anxiety problems. Whether a person experiences embarrassment as fear of others or as an altruistic concern about others, and whether a person expresses it with silence or with nervous laughter, also vary around the world's cultures. A person's sex and national origin may also influence whether shyness will cause tremendous shame and suffering or may be worn as a badge of virtue and pride.

Considering the role of culture in social anxiety also goes beyond a mere travelogue of exotic curiosities. Modern Western society is increasingly ambiguous in its rules, appearance oriented, and anonymous, with growing pressures to meet unattainable ideals of social attractiveness and performance. These trends feed feelings of inadequacy, embarrassment, social alienation, and withdrawal. It is possible that we are simply becoming more aware of some age-old frailties, although a more ominous possibility is that social phobia will become a growing public health problem of the twenty-first century. In any case, a better understanding of the cultural pressures on the individual may help us to meet these challenges.

IV

SOME OTHER FACES OF FEAR

12

STAGE FRIGHT, STARS, AND REAL PEOPLE

I had four minutes to be perfect and there were 3 billion people watching me on TV.

Madonna, explaining her trembling hands
while performing at the Academy Awards

No understanding of social anxiety could be complete without considering those who appear to be most free of social anxiety—professional performers. These people choose to earn their living in the one place where a having a social anxiety attack would be most natural, onstage. They seem to thrive on the thrill of it.

Nonperformers experience considerable trepidation at the mere thought of facing a large audience. This is not surprising, considering that we are "built" for more one-on-one or small group encounters, which made up the vast majority of social presentations over evolutionary history. When an animal attracted the rapt attention of a large group, it was usually a group of predators eyeing dinner.

Human audiences, too, have a long tradition of preying on performers. Where else in life is it ever considered acceptable for an observer to openly groan at or even heckle the performance of another? Not during a business presentation . . . or a first date. And when the stage is a playing field, the price of admission includes free license to berate athletic performers. For the audience, there is anonymity and safety

117

in numbers, a diffusion of responsibility for unkind behavior. For the exposed athlete, however, it ought to feel like the ultimate risk.

HOW PERFORMERS DO IT

So how do performers do it? People who dread the spotlight might assume that performers belong to some other species that experiences no anxiety, but such is not the case. In fact, having butterflies or jitters before some public presentations is a nearly universal experience. Professional performers cope with their fears by using techniques that could prove equally useful for Harry when giving his toast.

For one thing, performers often harness their nervous energy to enhance the quality of their performances. The veteran actor Carroll O'Connor has stated, "A professional actor has a kind of tension. . . . The amateur is thrown by it, but the professional needs it." Stevie Nicks, former lead singer of the rock group Fleetwood Mac, has also commented on that mix of fear and excitement: "If I wasn't really nervous before I walk onstage, I'd be really worried." For most pros, nervous energy gets channeled into the work at hand, and anxiety settles down once they are into their performances.

Performing arts psychologist Glenn D. Wilson has pointed out that it is not just the experience of anxiety but also the *timing* of anxiety that lead to success or failure on stage. While nearly all performers experience a gradual increase in apprehension before a performance, more successful ones reach their peak anxiety about an hour *before* the performance, rather than *during* it. This parallels the results of studies of parachutists showing that experienced parachutists are most nervous prior to the jump, while beginners are most frightened during the jump. The early peakers, whether they be parachutists or actors, are eventually able to focus on the performance itself and even to enjoy it. Those who peak later fare worse, of course, especially if during their late-peaking anxiety they forget their lines (or worse yet, forget to release their parachute lines).

Performers also cope by immersing themselves in their tasks, which tends to draw concentration away from their fears. Because the work of playing a role or a piece of music often requires total concentration, it is natural for the audience and a performer's extraneous fears to recede into the back of the mind. As time passes during a performance the situation loses its novelty, the performer's worst fears have not come to pass, and the anxiety weakens. In the language of psychology, habituation occurs.

The same sort of habituation that occurs over the course of a single

performance also tends to occur over the course of a performing career. With repeated exposure to a feared situation such as performing,
performers feel the fear gradually lessen. Some performers struggle
with anxiety early in their professional lives, when they are likely to
suffer the most rejections, but gain confidence as they become established and successful.

WHEN STAGE FRIGHT REACHES THE STARS

A relatively uncommon but remarkable exception is when this nervousness, instead of fading with time and experience, erupts into
persistent stage fright. Its typical symptoms are familiar to any
anxious public speaker: butterflies in the stomach, heart palpitations, sweating, trembling, and confusion.

Full-blown stage fright is a performer's worst nightmare. For
twenty-seven years, Barbra Streisand's problems with stage fright prevented her from singing in public. Despite her millions of adoring
fans and her secure place as a legend in popular music, Streisand
came to be obsessed with the idea that she might make humiliating
mistakes if she tried to perform again.

The traumatic moment that ignited this fear occurred during a free
concert in New York City's Central Park in 1967. Streisand forgot
the words to several songs, and she was visibly shaken. She redirected
her career to the more controllable medium of film, in which her
image could be reshot, cut, and otherwise massaged in the studio
before she presented it to the public. Twenty-seven years later, on the
eve of her comeback performance in Las Vegas, she explained the
origins of her stage fright to a reporter: "I forgot the words in front
of a hundred and twenty-five thousand people, and I wasn't cute about
it or anything . . . I was shocked; I was terrified. It prevented me from
performing for all these years."

The list of performers who have publicly acknowledged their battles
with stage fright reads like a celebrity Hall of Fame. Jerry Garcia,
former leader of the rock group The Grateful Dead, struggled with
stage fright throughout his career. Due to his social anxiety, Garcia
very rarely spoke to the audience between songs, even though his
fans showered him with cultlike unconditional love and devotion. The
esteemed British actress Glenda Jackson had publicly disclosed that
she suffers heart palpitations and worries she will be unable to perform
in the minutes prior to a stage performance. Acclaim and awards have

done nothing to allay her fears: "I suppose it's that the more you do, the more you realize how painfully easy it is to be lousy and how very difficult it is to be good." Even Mikhail Baryshnikov, while reigning for years as the world's premier male ballet dancer, would become consumed with nervousness prior to a performance. "Always I have butterflies in stomach," he confessed at the height of his success. World famous cellist Pablo Casals acknowledged that throughout his career he struggled with stage fright, even losing his grip on his bow during an important concert as a result of anxiety-induced sweating.

Theater legend Sir Laurence Olivier recounted in his autobiography a prolonged bout with stage fright that struck in the prime of his career. He was acting at the National Theater, which had recently opened in London with Olivier as director. The problem began with an "appalling thought"—that he might be too tired to remember his lines.

> My courage sank, and with each succeeding minute it became less possible to resist this horror. My cue came, and I went on to that state where I knew with grim certainty I would not be capable of remaining more than a few minutes. . . . My voice had started to fade, my throat closed up and the audience was beginning to go giddily round. . . . With unusual inaudibility, owing to my tightly clenched teeth, I somehow got on with the play. . . .

Olivier recalled that what he referred to as "the disease" continued to torment him for a full five years. During a run of *Othello,* he feared that he would not be able to stay onstage alone, noting that "everyone who had scenes with me had to know what was going on, in order to be able to cope in case of trouble."

Another venue where stars have been hobbled by performance anxiety is the sports arena. Former New York Mets catcher Mackey Sasser endured a humiliating season in which he developed self-conscious fears of misthrowing the baseball back to the mound after each pitch. Fans would hoot and howl at the nervous habits he had developed: pumping, double-pumping, and even triple-pumping his throwing arm before releasing the ball. A similar problem, with career-ending consequences, befell baseball hero Steve Blass, star pitcher for the Pittsburgh Pirates. After completing record-breaking seasons as a World Series hero in 1971 and an All-Star Team member in 1972, Blass developed a crippling fear of being watched as he pitched in 1973. Although he would throw perfect strikes during practice when no one was watching, Blass was unable to throw the ball near the plate during a live ball game. Due to this problem, he was forced to retire from baseball in 1974 at the age of thirty-two.

HOW CAN VETERANS BE SO VULNERABLE?

It may seem surprising that veteran performers can be toppled by the same jitters that commonly stymie beginners. Why do performers at the peak of their careers remain vulnerable to crippling performance anxiety? There are at least several factors involved. First there is the obvious: The risk of embarrassment or humiliation is always present when a performer is scrutinized by an audience. This potential for failure is part and parcel of the spontaneity that makes live performance so vibrant and appealing to watch. All the experience in the world cannot eliminate the possibility of a blooper.

In fact, for the well-established successful performer, the stakes may feel far higher. Many star performers have been successful precisely because they are so *driven* to get a positive response from their audience. Performers may become obsessed with the opinion of their public, despite the danger of depending on something so fickle. The accomplished performer's own formidable pressures to succeed are now multiplied by the pressures of fans, agents, and producers. And the media that creates the trappings of superstardom is always ready to destroy its creation. Huge expectations are raised by a star's success, and they must be met—or else.

The nature of a creative performance itself may increase vulnerability to a host of emotions, including stage fright. To achieve peak ability in art or sport, performers often need to follow their emotions, to let emotion inspire them. The adrenaline flows, but if creativity is said to be 10 percent inspiration and 90 percent perspiration, a good part of the latter is often the cold sweat of anxiety. The same creative energy that feeds a winning performance may get diverted into the frightening arousal of panic.

STAGE FRIGHT SOLUTIONS

Many stage performers turn to medication in order to control stage fright. The prescription medications most widely used for this purpose are beta-blockers, which block the effects of adrenaline and thereby reduce distracting symptoms such as a pounding heart, shaky hands, and clammy palms. We discuss beta-blocker medications and the controversy over their widespread use by performers in chapter 19. Cognitive-behavioral therapy, which we discuss in chapter 18, has also been shown to be effective in reducing performance anxiety in musicians.

Many successful performers ultimately find their own ways to cope with their bouts of stage fright. In her 1994 comeback tour, Streisand maintained tremendous control over each performance, using Tele-PrompTers as cue cards for every song lyric and for her between-song banter. Nothing was left unplanned. Nonetheless, as is true for many sufferers with irrational performance fears, superpreparation only partially allayed Streisand's apprehension before each show: "I get sick to my stomach before I go on," she confessed to reporters. Yet go on she did, completing one of the most successful concert tours in history.

What, then, is the explanation for the transformation from fearful avoider to reborn star performer? Streisand made a decision to begin a step-by-step program of exposure to her fear, stage performance, which enabled her to begin to accumulate positive experiences. She tested the waters with a few "warm-up" shows in Las Vegas that eventually led to a national tour, culminating in an extremely successful performance in front of a large television audience. The gradual accumulation of positive responses to her shows promoted a fundamental shift in Streisand's thinking: "We were talking about how far I'd come from Vegas, when I had to take Lomotil [an antidiarrhea drug] and lost weight and sleep. I thought I really would disappoint people, that I wasn't good enough. Soon in my growth process, I've come to realize I'm pretty good. I don't know why I'm good, but I know that I am good. And now that I have more sense of that, the imperfections are OK. Whoever I am is good enough to be there."

Perhaps these were the very words that served Streisand as silently spoken responses to her fear while she was onstage ("I know that I am good"). It seems she was able to shift from focusing on the possibility of making a mistake (which always remained present) and fearing a catastrophic negative reaction from the audience (which she could not directly control) to focusing on her own basic capabilities, which she truly believed in. This new "self-talk" may have displaced her old "I'll flub my lines and be humiliated," the type of thinking that had fueled her avoidance of the stage for twenty-seven years. In turn, renewed confidence gradually displaced her fear.

Of course, you don't have to be a superstar performing in front of a packed house at Madison Square Garden to experience stage fright. Small and relatively unimportant performances can create the same intensity of fear reaction. Singing in the church choir, telling a joke to a few friends, or even just introducing yourself to a group of strangers can set off the same kind of panic.

SAM, FEARFUL PART-TIME GUITARIST

Although most performers weather stage fright without ever understanding its exact origins, in some cases the foundations for stage fright seem to have been laid early in life. Sam climbed to the top of his high school's tennis team, performed solos with a jazz band, and was elected president of the Student Council. Sam's parents, however, were unimpressed by his extracurricular achievements. In an effort to encourage him to pursue the secure career of medicine, they praised Sam only when he got good grades or talked about the possibility of becoming a doctor, and they pooh-poohed his potential as a musician. Sam continued to pursue his music, but, conforming to his parents' wishes, he majored in science in college and got accepted into a prestigious medical school.

It was in medical school that Sam's particular social fear began to grow. Although Sam continued to perform in a jazz band, with the demands of school limiting his practice time, he felt as if his musical efforts had become an embarrassment. While he had never before experienced more than slight preperformance jitters, he became increasingly preoccupied with fears that he would panic onstage and humiliate himself.

To the other band members, Sam's fears seemed ludicrous. His musical abilities remained outstanding—and all the more remarkable for someone in the middle of medical school. But Sam felt different. Although many of his classmates had dropped extracurricular interests completely, for Sam it was excellence in music that made him feel good about himself and that made the rote memorization of the classroom tolerable. To forfeit that musical excellence for medicine seemed akin to letting his spirit die.

Fears of stage fright left Sam a mess in the days prior to a performance. He had difficulty concentrating on his studies, and nervousness even began to interfere with his clinical work, where he had trouble listening to patients' complaints or focusing on taking a blood pressure. By his third year in medical school, Sam had become depressed over his inability to overcome the fear, so he sidestepped the problem by quitting music altogether.

It wasn't until he had completed his residency program in ophthalmology several years later that Sam began the process of trying to understand his problem. He began to disclose snippets of his losing battle with stage fright to one of us (L.W.), whom he had befriended at the hospital where he worked. During lunch and coffee breaks at the hospital cafeteria, I pointed out some of the inconsistencies in Sam's thinking about stage performance: "On the one hand you tell me that you're an accomplished musician, yet you often tell yourself that you're a lousy musician. So, which one is true? Are you good or lousy?" Sam began to recognize that he had been stymied by his perfectionism. He was also taken by an idea I had suggested as one of the roots of this perfectionism: that he felt a need to star in music in order to disprove his parents' old criticisms.

With some encouragement, Sam began once again to dabble in performing, with the added proviso that he "talk to himself" realistically about his own abilities ("I'm really good enough to enjoy this and to give others pleasure"), particularly in the days and moments before a performance. Sam began to play guitar in "low-pressure" places such as the home of a friend or a local coffeehouse. From time to time he would complain over coffee that he still wasn't sure that he was a good enough musician and that maybe he was deluding himself. I wouldn't buy it: "This old story really isn't that interesting. If criticism is what you want, go talk to your parents about your music. Otherwise, tell me and tell yourself what you like about music. . . ." Sam smiled and suggested that if he had really wanted to analyze himself he would have gone into psychiatry instead of ophthalmology.

RACHEL—REVERSE STAGE FRIGHT

Most people with social fears of any type would rather be anywhere but onstage. That makes all the more remarkable the performer for whom the stage is a refuge from the social phobia she suffers when out of a role. Rachel, a twenty-three-year-old actress living in New York, had no problems whatsoever with stage fright: "I would stand on the auditioning line eating a pastrami sandwich dripping with cole-slaw while everyone else was pacing around or sucking down Pepto-Bismol." For Rachel, social anxiety would engulf her outside the theater—at parties or dealing with authority figures at the Actors' Equity union, where she would become nervous asking for information about medical benefits.

Acting onstage was a welcome escape from the social fears of Rachel's everyday life. As she saw it, acting allowed her to become a confident person through taking on roles that were very different from her real self. Her role relieved her of the responsibility for her own behavior. She could act brash without offending any "real" person. If the role called for it, she could say the "wrong thing" without embarrassing her real self. Rachel knew she could act, but she doubted that people would appreciate her for who she really was.

Rachel had also adopted the role of the actor to help her cope with her real-life social fears. Acting the part of a self-confident extrovert, or "faking it," seemed to help her get started at a party or when dealing with authority figures. She found this maneuver temporarily liberating, but she also feared that it wouldn't be helpful in the long run. If she spent her whole life playacting, just who was she anyway?

In therapy, Rachel came to recognize that immersing herself in a make-believe persona was a way of avoiding her fears, almost in the same way as if she were to avoid parties or authority figures altogether. As an avoider, she missed out on opportunities to disprove her worst fears. So when people told her she had been the life of a party, Rachel could dismiss her success as "just acting," and she could maintain the belief that in real life she was terribly boring.

She began to experiment with putting her "real" self on the line by telling true stories about herself and trying not to censor her own feelings so much. As she noted that others, on the whole, seemed to respond positively to her new honesty, her self-confidence grew. She discovered that her make-believe outgoing persona had not been just a figment of her acting imagination. Instead it also had been a real part of herself that she had avoided accepting. As she took more chances, revealing herself, her fear decreased, it became easier for Rachel to be herself, and her self naturally became more outgoing in turn.

13

SEXUAL ANXIETY AND SHYNESS

Man is a mind betrayed, not served, by his organs.

Edmond and Jules DeGoncort, 1861

Blushing is the color of virtue.

Diogenes, fourth century B.C.

For the person with social anxiety, developing a sexual relationship can present multiple problems. Shy people tend to have difficulty meeting others and initiating dates, and social anxiety can interfere with the open expression of feelings that moves a relationship toward emotional intimacy. Because they date less often, socially anxious people tend to be inexperienced, which further increases their anxiety. In regard to sexual activity, psychologist Phillip Zimbardo, surveying college students in the 1970s, reported that 37 percent of shy students had had sexual intercourse, compared to 62 percent of students who were not shy. Other studies have found that people with social anxiety are often troubled by lack of sexual desire as well, although they consider sex to be extremely important to their happiness. Even when socially anxious people do get involved in sexual relationships, they tend to find them less satisfying.

TODD'S STORY

One common cause of sexual dissatisfaction in socially anxious people is performance anxiety. At age thirty-five, Todd felt he had finally met the woman of his dreams. Lena was very attractive, smart, fun to be with, and from their first date she made it clear that she was equally excited about him. After two months of seeing each other a few times each week, they were pretty comfortable with each other and they had been physically affectionate: holding hands, hugging, kissing, fondling, and massaging each other. The only thing about this relationship that scared the daylights out of Todd was also what he longed for the most: the prospect of making love to Lena.

Todd feared that he would not be able to maintain an erection. He had experienced this problem with some, but not all, of the other women he had been with. It seemed to occur with the women he had cared for the most, and he would inevitably feel devastated. The more important it was for everything to go right, the more likely his penis was to refuse to cooperate, mocking his desires. Twice before he had ended promising relationships rather than face persistent humiliation. This time Todd sought professional help.

It turned out that although Todd was not generally self-conscious with people, he had experienced a pattern of anxiety problems in situations where he felt he was being evaluated. In high school band he had declined opportunities to play solo trombone parts due to fears of being embarrassed by "choking." He stayed away from theater after muffing a line in his sixth grade class play. As far back as first grade he had been reluctant to raise his hand in class, but he had learned to overcome that one. These difficulties had stayed on the edges of Todd's life for the most part, hardly causing any real interference. Now things were different.

Before determining that performance anxiety was the cause of Todd's difficulties, it was essential to rule out physical causes, which increasingly have been shown to play a role in many cases of impotence. In Todd's case, a physical cause seemed unlikely for several reasons: In addition to his history of other performance fears, his ability to have an erection varied depending on how he felt about the woman. In the absence of a woman, he regularly woke up with normal spontaneous erections, and he was able to have normal erections when masturbating. He was young, otherwise healthy, and he wasn't taking any medications that might have been responsible for the problem.

TREATMENT OF SEXUAL
PERFORMANCE ANXIETY

In the 1970s, sex researchers Masters and Johnson called attention to performance anxiety as a cause of erectile problems in men and orgasm difficulty in women. They noted that in many such cases, the distraction of fearful thoughts about being unable to please a partner led to decreased sexual performance. When performance anxiety seemed to be the problem, it responded fairly readily to straightforward behavioral remedies. These techniques involved teaching sufferers and their partners to reduce the pressure to perform. At the same time, patients learned to focus on the experience of their own pleasure, rather than obsessively focusing on pleasing a partner.

More recently, the sex researchers' earlier beliefs that performance anxiety causes inability to sustain an erection were challenged by scientific studies showing that a moderate level of anxiety often seems to actually enhance sexual arousal in both men and women. Psychologist David Barlow was able to disentangle this paradox with a series of studies done in the 1980s. These studies showed that men with sexual performance problems showed several key differences from other men, including how they responded to anxiety.

First, the men with trouble sustaining erections tended to underestimate the strength of their erections. This was studied in a laboratory setting in which subjects viewed an erotic film while the size of their erections was measured by a mechanical device. The subjects were unable to view themselves. The troubled men were more likely to sense only a weak erection when it was actually strong. The same kind of underestimation of their own physiological sexual arousal seems to be present in women with sexual functioning problems.

In another study, men viewed an erotic film while being distracted by hearing a nonsexual passage read from a novel. The distraction tended to reduce the arousal of the healthy men, but not that of the troubled men. The two groups of men also differed in their reactions to the behavior of a sexual partner. A film which portrayed a sexual partner as more "turned on" tended to increase arousal for the healthy men, but it decreased arousal and raised anxiety for the troubled men. Finally, when men were told they might receive a mild electric shock while watching the erotic film, troubled men became less aroused, but healthy men were actually more aroused.

Barlow's findings support the idea that fear of failing their partners causes men with sexual performance anxiety to perform worse. Underestimation of the true quality of their erections may add to their anxiety, mild anxiety is not a turn-on for them (as it may be for normal men), and the fear of failing to meet their partners' expectations becomes a self-fulfilling prophecy. Bad experiences lead to the old vicious cycle of avoidance, increased fears, and worse performance. If these men can take their minds off their fears, such as through distraction, their performance will improve.

Todd's Treatment

The treatment of Todd's sexual performance anxiety was guided by some of the principles of this recent research. One goal was for Todd to reduce his performance pressure. After several sessions in which we discussed the pros and cons of some ways in which he might approach this, Todd decided he would have little to lose at this point by telling his girlfriend, Lena, about his problem, as she must have already realized something was amiss. It turned out she had been wondering if he had some more serious hang-up about sex, and she was pleased to know that he cared enough about her to reveal his problem. Lena offered to try to help him overcome the problem, in the process becoming a key support instead of a secret adversary.

To further reduce his performance pressures, Todd and Lena agreed that they would forgo sexual intercourse for several weeks. She told him some things that he could do to please her sexually, and he planned to focus on the pleasurable sensations he experienced when she touched him, rather than on fears of whether he could perform. Todd was instructed to accept that he might get fears about whether he was having an erection, and that rather than dwell on them or fight them, he should just let them naturally pass as he returned his attention to pleasurable sensations he was experiencing.

After a few weeks, the couple was gradually feeling more comfortable together. Shortly thereafter, however, they reported that they had been unable to follow the plan. They had gotten carried away and had intercourse. Several times. Without difficulty or major anxiety. These are the failures that make therapy so rewarding.

Before we congratulate ourselves over the progress we have made in treatment, it's worth recognizing that not much in this world is truly new. In 1786, at a time when impotence was erroneously believed to be caused by excessive masturbation in childhood, an early case of behavior therapy was described by John Hunter, surgeon to St. George's Hospital, London, and to George III:

A gentlemen told me, that he had lost his powers ... After above an hour's investigation of the case, I made out the following facts: that he had at unnecessary times strong erections, which showed that he had naturally this power; that the erections were accompanied with desire ... but that there was still a defect somewhere, which I supposed to be from the mind. I inquired if all women were alike to him, his answer was no; some women he could have connection with, as well as ever .. it appeared that there was but one woman that produced this inability, and that it arose from a desire to perform the act with this woman well; which desire produced in the mind a doubt, or fear of the want of success, which was the cause of the inability of performing the act ... I told him that he might be cured ... He was to go to bed to this woman, but first promise to himself, that he would not have any connection with her, for six nights ... About a fortnight after he told me that this resolution had produced such a total alteration in the state of his mind, that the power soon took place, for instead of going to bed with the fear of inability, he went with fears that he should be possessed with too much desire, too much power ... and when he had once broke the spell, the mind and powers went on together; his mind never returning to its former state.

WHY SEX IS A POTENT TRIGGER OF ANXIETY

It is not surprising that sex is a focal point for problems in people with a tendency to have social fears of being evaluated. Looking back through evolutionary history, in most species of social animals we see that social fear and lower social status tend to reduce an individual's opportunities to mate. But we have yet to hear of a sheep or monkey with performance anxiety. It takes the bigger, sexier brains of humans to be able to inject psychology and self-consciousness into the sex act itself.

Sex provokes anxiety because it is so important to people. This is evident throughout our society, as sex appeal is used to sell everything from toothpaste to power tools. Because sex is the most intimate of all forms of expression, failure or rejection in this area of life cannot easily be dismissed. The audience is usually only one person, but this person's opinion tends to carry great weight. And most people have their first sexual experiences during adolescence or early adulthood, around the age when they are most vulnerable to social anxiety.

In addition to the importance of sex, its novelty also tends to provoke anxiety. Having sex with a new partner is for most people relatively uncommon, compared to, say, having a conversation with a new acquaintance. Also, the act of sex breaks all sorts of taboos that in other situations would trigger unthinkable embarrassment or shame: exposing one's naked body, being touched in private places, experiencing pleasures that one may have been taught are shameful. In some cases, anxiety about sex may carry important Freudian baggage, such as unconscious fears of being castrated as punishment for forbidden sexual and aggressive wishes.

As with other social anxieties, perfectionistic expectations contribute to anxiety about sex. Because discussing sex is either difficult or prohibited for many people, sex is particularly likely to be the subject of unrealistic attitudes. When it is discussed, information is often distorted, as when adolescents embellish their experiences bragging to peers, or in Hollywood films. The latter most commonly depict a couple with perfect bodies reaching simultaneous orgasm after a few frames of lovemaking. Men "learn" that they should be able to perform on demand, and repeatedly; women "learn" that they should always have an orgasm during intercourse, after foreplay that consists of one passionate kiss and embrace.

Men are more likely than women to feel humiliated by problems with sexual performance in particular, because failure to maintain an erection is impossible to conceal or ignore. But these men's partners suffer as well, wondering if they are somehow to blame, if they are not desirable enough, or if the man is not attracted to them. Fears of embarrassment may mingle with other unrelated disturbing feelings, such as having mixed feelings about a partner, concerns over the adequacy of a birth control method, or concerns about protection from sexually transmitted disease.

SEXUAL SHYNESS

Women may be more likely than men to feel shame about their sexual activity and more likely to be embarrassed about expressing sexual desire or pleasure, or about exposing their bodies. It is likely that such sexual modesty results from a combination of biological influences, which may tend to steer women away from situations that could result in unwanted pregnancy; psychological influences, such as women's greater self-consciousness in general; and cultural influences. The latter include traditional beliefs of most of the major religions that limit women's expression of sexuality and lead to shame over sexual desires. Another cultural factor is society's obsession with ideals of feminine beauty, as evidenced in the advertising, fashion, cosmetics, and weight loss industries. The inability of most women to attain these ideals contributes to women's feelings of self-consciousness and embarrassment about their bodies.

In Western society the origins of shame over the human body and sexuality go back to Genesis and the Garden of Eden. After violating God's commandment not to eat from the tree of knowledge, Adam and Eve became self-conscious of their nakedness for the first time, and they hid from God. Their shame over disobeying God was instantaneously associated with shame over their own nakedness.

Just as women have been taught for centuries to experience shame and embarrassment over their bodies, they have been taught that expressing such embarrassment or sexual modesty is desirable, a sign of feminine virtue. Prior to the twentieth century, blushing was widely believed to have been specially designed by the Creator to serve as a sign to others that sacred rules were being violated. So a woman who failed to blush and display embarrassment over nudity or sexuality was thought to reveal a lack of moral character. Ironically, some of the same male writers who hailed the blush as a sign of feminine virtue also found it incredibly attractive. In 1774, Dr. John Gregory went so far as to contend that Nature has "forced" men to love a blushing young woman. In spite of the sexual revolution in recent decades, these deeply embedded beliefs about sex linger on.

V

An Owner's Manual for Social Anxiety

14

TAKING MEASURE OF SOCIAL ANXIETY

If having some social anxiety is perfectly normal, but having too much can interfere with everyday functioning and can signal the disorder of social phobia, how do you know where you stand? Some simple tests can help determine whether your own social anxiety is a problem you ought to address. In this chapter we present several questionnaires that assess different aspects of social anxiety. Researchers have found these questionnaires to be useful for measuring social anxiety and its effects.

BEFORE YOU TRY THE TESTS

Taking a social anxiety self-test may be helpful in several ways: A test can show how you compare in terms of social anxiety to the general public and to people who have a clinical diagnosis of social phobia. Finding that your score falls within the common range can be reassuring. Alternatively, discovering that you score in the same ballpark as people with social phobia can alert you to a potential problem.

A test can also help identify specific problem areas that are sometimes difficult to notice in everyday life. For some people, avoiding particular social situations, such as public speaking or speaking to authority figures, becomes so routine that they don't even realize the avoidance is limiting their lives. Others feel troubled in a general way but may not be able to pinpoint the problem area. Answering some pertinent questions can provide a new perspective, however, and recognizing a social anxiety problem is the first step to mastering it.

People with social anxiety are especially curious, not surprisingly, to know how they compare to others. After all, a key feature of social phobia is excessive fear of failing to measure up to the standards of other people. Because the tests we have selected have all been previously published and used by researchers studying social anxiety, we have been able to list some published "norms" for different groups on each test, which makes it easier to estimate where your own anxiety fits in the spectrum.

It is important, however, to recognize the limitations of these tests. A test score alone cannot determine whether you have a problem with social anxiety. For each test there is some overlap of the scores of people with anxiety problems and those without. What is "normal" for you also depends on your age, sex, and other factors in your life. For example, a score on the Personal Report of Confidence as a Public Speaker may be irrelevant to someone who has no need or desire to do any public speaking. So tests may help you clarify your situation, but they cannot substitute for common sense or for a comprehensive evaluation by a mental health professional.

TESTING YOUR FEARS OF INTERACTING

One difficulty in trying to measure social anxiety problems on a single scale is that these problems take different forms in different people. For example, some people fear going to parties and meeting new people, while others might not mind attending a party but dread the idea of giving a talk in public. Some people are concerned that they will perform a task badly in front of an audience, while others fear the audience will notice them blush. The Interaction Anxiousness Scale, developed by psychologist Mark Leary, examines a variety of anxious feelings in a variety of social situations.

Interaction Anxiousness Scale

Read each item carefully and decide the degree to which the statement is characteristic or true of you. Then place a number from 1 to 5 in the correct space according to the following scale.

1 = The statement is *not* at all characteristic of me.
2 = The statement is *slightly* characteristic of me.
3 = The statement is *moderately* characteristic of me.
4 = The statement is *very* characteristic of me.
5 = The statement is *extremely* characteristic of me.

_____ 1. I often feel nervous even in casual get-togethers.

_____ 2. I usually feel uncomfortable when I am in a group of people I don't know.

_____ 3. I am usually not at ease when speaking to a member of the opposite sex.

_____ 4. I get nervous when I must talk to a teacher or boss.

_____ 5. Parties often make me feel anxious and uncomfortable.

_____ 6. I am probably more shy in social interactions than most people.

_____ 7. I sometimes feel tense when talking to people of my own sex if I don't know them very well.

_____ 8. I would be nervous if I was being interviewed for a job.

_____ 9. I wish I had more confidence in social situations.

_____ 10. I often feel anxious in social situations.

_____ 11. In general, I am a shy person.

_____ 12. I often feel nervous when talking to an attractive member of the opposite sex.

_____ 13. I often feel nervous when calling someone I don't know very well on the telephone.

_____ 14. I get nervous when I speak to someone in a position of authority.

_____ 15. I usually feel nervous around other people, even people who are quite different from myself.

_____ Total Score, Interaction Anxiousness Scale

Interpreting Your Score—A study of college students found that those seeking help for social anxiety problems scored an average of 55 on this test, and a random group of students averaged a score of 38.

In addition to noting how your total score compares with the scores of these reference groups, your score on an individual item may be informative. Are there particular situations that create a high degree of discomfort or anxiety? For example, is your anxiety focused on interacting with people of the opposite sex? Your responses to specific items may guide you to particular areas you want work on.

TESTING FEAR AND AVOIDANCE OF SITUATIONS

The Liebowitz Social Anxiety Scale is also helpful for identifying which sorts of social and performance situations trigger anxiety and avoidance. This rating scale was developed by researchers at Columbia University to study the treatment of social phobia. For each situation listed on the scale, record two numbers: one that indicates how fearful or anxious you typically feel in that situation, and a second that indicates how likely you are to avoid it. If a particular situation occurs only rarely for you, imagine how anxious you *would* be and how likely you *would* be to avoid the situation if it did come up. Calculate your overall total score by adding up the numbers from each column and then adding together these fear and avoidance subtotals (the highest possible score is 144, the lowest is 0).

Liebowitz Social Anxiety Scale

Rate how much fear or anxiety you typically would experience in each situation and how often you would avoid the situation, using the key below:

FEAR OR ANXIETY	AVOIDANCE
0 = None	0 = Never
1 = Mild	1 = Occasionally
2 = Moderate	2 = Often
3 = Severe	3 = Usually

	FEAR OR ANXIETY	AVOIDANCE
1. Telephoning in public	0 1 2 3	0 1 2 3
2. Participating in small groups	0 1 2 3	0 1 2 3
3. Eating in public places	0 1 2 3	0 1 2 3
4. Drinking with others in public places	0 1 2 3	0 1 2 3
5. Talking to people in authority	0 1 2 3	0 1 2 3
6. Acting, performing, or giving a talk in front of an audience	0 1 2 3	0 1 2 3
7. Going to a party	0 1 2 3	0 1 2 3

	FEAR OR ANXIETY	AVOIDANCE
8. Working while being observed	0 1 2 3	0 1 2 3
9. Writing while being observed	0 1 2 3	0 1 2 3
10. Calling someone you don't know very well	0 1 2 3	0 1 2 3
11. Talking with people you don't know very well	0 1 2 3	0 1 2 3
12. Meeting strangers	0 1 2 3	0 1 2 3
13. Urinating in a public bathroom	0 1 2 3	0 1 2 3
14. Entering a room when others are already seated	0 1 2 3	0 1 2 3
15. Being the center of attention	0 1 2 3	0 1 2 3
16. Speaking up at a meeting	0 1 2 3	0 1 2 3
17. Taking a test	0 1 2 3	0 1 2 3
18. Expressing disagreement or disapproval to people you don't know very well	0 1 2 3	0 1 2 3
19. Looking at people you don't know very well in the eyes	0 1 2 3	0 1 2 3
20. Giving a report to a group	0 1 2 3	0 1 2 3
21. Trying to pick up someone	0 1 2 3	0 1 2 3
22. Returning goods to a store	0 1 2 3	0 1 2 3
23. Giving a party	0 1 2 3	0 1 2 3
24. Resisting a high-pressure salesperson	0 1 2 3	0 1 2 3

Subtotal Scores: Fear or Anxiety_____ + Avoidance_____ =
_____ Total Score, Social Anxiety Scale

Interpreting Your Score—In research studies, persons seeking treatment for social phobia have averaged overall total scores of about 70 on the Liebowitz Social Anxiety Scale, with most scores within a range of 35 to 100.

While a total score above 35 indicates a good chance of a problem with social anxiety, a low score needs to be examined more closely before drawing any conclusions. This is because even with a low score, individual items with scores of 2 or 3 can point out particular areas that may be problematic.

This scale has also been used to measure improvement during treatment. When improvement occurs gradually, it may show up on a rating scale before it becomes more obvious. In research studies, people with social phobia who are treated with effective medication or a cognitive-behavioral therapy show about a 50 percent improvement, as a rough average, in their overall score after two to three months (see chapters 18 and 19 for more information on treatments). You may want to repeat the Liebowitz Social Anxiety Scale after you have completed a few months of treatment or after trying the self-help program we outline in chapter 15.

TESTING THE IMPACT OF SOCIAL ANXIETY ON YOUR LIFE

Another test developed by researchers at Columbia University is the Liebowitz Disability Self-Rating Scale. It was designed to measure how much social anxiety interferes with a person's functioning in everyday life. The questionnaire yields two types of total scores: The "current" disability score is most useful, as it reflects how much your anxiety problem has been interfering with your life in the past two weeks. For social anxiety problems that were more severe in the past, the "lifetime" disability score reflects how much they interfered with your life when the social anxiety was at its worst.

People tend to underestimate the extent to which social anxiety has affected their lives. To complete this test accurately, it can help to consider this additional question before answering each question about whether anxiety has limited your functioning: "If I were free of social anxiety problems, would anything be different for me in this area of my life?" Try to be honest with yourself.

Liebowitz Disability Self-Rating Scale

How much does your emotional problem (social fear and avoidance) limit your ability to do each of the following? Circle 0, 1, 2, or 3 for each question.

	Problem does not limit me at all	Problem limits me slightly	Problem limits me a moderate extent	Problem limits me severely
1. Mainly being in a good mood when things are going well?				
During the past 2 weeks:	0	1	2	3
Lifetime/When I was at my worst:	0	1	2	3
2. Going as far in school as my money and intelligence permit?				
During the past 2 weeks:	0	1	2	3
Lifetime/When I was at my worst:	0	1	2	3
3. Keeping a job (housework or work outside of the home) that allows me to work to my highest ability?				
During the past 2 weeks:	0	1	2	3
Lifetime/When I was at my worst:	0	1	2	3
4. Having mostly comfortable interactions with the members of my family?				
During the past 2 weeks:	0	1	2	3
Lifetime/When I was at my worst:	0	1	2	3
5. Having a satisfying romantic/intimate relationship?				
During the past 2 weeks:	0	1	2	3
Lifetime/When I was at my worst:	0	1	2	3
6. Having at least a few close friends and a small group of acquaintances?				
During the past 2 weeks:	0	1	2	3
Lifetime/When I was at my worst:	0	1	2	3
7. Pursuing hobbies and other interests (e.g., religion, sports, etc.)?				
During the past 2 weeks:	0	1	2	3
Lifetime/When I was at my worst:	0	1	2	3

	Problem does not limit me at all	*Problem limits me slightly*	*Problem limits me a moderate extent*	*Problem limits me severely*
8. Taking care of personal shopping, household chores and personal hygiene (e.g., bathing, showering, brushing your teeth)?				
During the past 2 weeks:	0	1	2	3
Lifetime/When I was at my worst:	0	1	2	3

Disability Scale
Current Total Score_____
Lifetime Total Score_____

Interpreting Your Score—One research study used this scale to compare adults who were free of anxiety problems to adults who were diagnosed with social phobia. The nonanxious group averaged less than 1 on both "Current Total" and "Lifetime Total" scores. The subjects with social phobia, however, averaged scores of about 8 on the current scale and 12 on the lifetime scale. One reason that the current scores were lower than lifetime scores for the social phobic subjects in the study was because most of them had already started treatment for their problem.

As with the previous scale, a score of 2 or 3 on an individual item may identify a problem area. Figuring out how seriously social anxiety interferes with functioning is often the most critical issue in determining whether a person's social anxiety is a significant problem.

TESTING YOUR CONFIDENCE AS A PUBLIC SPEAKER

For anxiety related to public speaking activities, such as giving a toast at a wedding, speaking up in class, or giving public speeches, this test can help measure the severity of the problem. The Personal Report of Confidence as a Speaker was originally developed in the 1940s as a research tool for studying communication skills. Years later it was modified, and it is now used to measure speech anxiety.

Personal Report of Confidence as a Speaker (PRCS)

For each item circle "True" or "False," whichever *best* represents your feelings associated with your most recent speech. Compute your total score by adding the scores (0 or 1) that go along with the answers you have circled.

1. I look forward to an opportunity to speak in public.
   True (0)   *False* (1)
2. My hands tremble when I try to handle objects on the platform.
   True (1)   *False* (0)
3. I am in constant fear of forgetting my speech.
   True (1)   *False* (0)
4. Audiences seem friendly when I address them.
   True (0)   *False* (1)
5. While preparing a speech I am in a constant state of anxiety.
   True (1)   *False* (0)
6. At the conclusion of a speech I feel that I have had a pleasant experience.
   True (0)   *False* (1)
7. I dislike using my body and voice expressively.
   True (1)   *False* (0)
8. My thoughts become confused and jumbled when I speak before an audience.
   True (1)   *False* (0)
9. I have no fear of facing an audience.
   True (0)   *False* (1)
10. Although I am nervous just before getting up, I soon forget my fears and enjoy the experience.
    True (0)   *False* (1)
11. I face the prospect of making a speech with complete confidence.
    True (0)   *False* (1)
12. I feel that I am in complete possession of myself while speaking.
    True (0)   *False* (1)
13. I prefer to have notes on the platform in case I forget my speech.
    True (1)   *False* (0)
14. I like to observe the reactions of my audience to my speech.
    True (0)   *False* (1)
15. Although I talk fluently with friends, I am at a loss for words on the platform.
    True (1)   *False* (0)

16. I feel relaxed and comfortable while speaking.
    True (0)   *False* (1)

17. Although I do not enjoy speaking in public, I do not particularly dread it.
    True (0)   *False* (1)

18. I always avoid speaking in public if possible.
    True (1)   *False* (0)

19. The faces of my audience are blurred when I look at them.
    True (1)   *False* (0)

20. I feel disgusted with myself after trying to address a group of people.
    True (1)   *False* (0)

21. I enjoy preparing a talk.
    True (0)   *False* (1)

22. My mind is clear when I face an audience.
    True (0)   *False* (1)

23. I am fairly fluent.
    True (0)   *False* (1)

24. I perspire and tremble just before getting up to speak.
    True (1)   *False* (0)

25. My posture feels strained and unnatural.
    True (1)   *False* (0)

26. I am fearful and tense all the while I am speaking before a group of people.
    True (1)   *False* (0)

27. I find the prospect of speaking mildly pleasant.
    True (0)   *False* (1)

28. It is difficult for me to search my mind calmly for the right words to express my thoughts.
    True (1)   *False* (0)

29. I am terrified at the thought of speaking before a group of people.
    True (1)   *False* (0)

30. I have a feeling of alertness while facing an audience.
    True (0)   *False* (1)

_____Total Score, Personal Report of Confidence as a Speaker

Interpreting Your Score—Studies with different groups of subjects have shown a wide range of scores on this scale. In a large study of college students enrolled in speech courses, one investigator found an average score of about 12, with 70 percent of the test takers scoring between 6 and 18. This average score may be a bit higher than the average for the general population, because students with fears of public speaking may be more likely to enroll in speech courses to overcome their fears. Scores above 18 are likely to reflect a problem with public speaking. Another study showed that people with no fear of public speaking scored an average of about 5, whereas people who considered themselves to have a public speaking phobia scored about 20 on average.

If you scored high in public speaking anxiety, you may want to reflect on whether your anxiety extends into areas beyond public speaking. In addition to this test, go back and look over your scores on the earlier tests of more general social anxiety.

TESTING YOUR CHILD'S SOCIAL FEARS

The Social Anxiety Scale for Children was designed for use with children of elementary school age (grades 2 through 6). It includes items about worrisome thinking ("I worry about being teased") and behavior ("I'm quiet when I'm with a group of kids"). Children can complete the form on their own, but those who need assistance in reading and understanding the questions can be helped by an adult.

Social Anxiety Scale for Children

1. I worry about doing something new in front of other kids.

0	1	2
Never True	*Sometimes True*	*Always True*

2. I worry about being teased.

0	1	2
Never True	*Sometimes True*	*Always True*

3. I feel shy around kids I don't know.

0	1	2
Never True	*Sometimes True*	*Always True*

4. I'm quiet when I'm with a group of kids.

0	1	2
Never True	*Sometimes True*	*Always True*

5. I worry about what other kids think of me.

0	1	2
Never True	*Sometimes True*	*Always True*

6. I feel that kids are making fun of me.

0	1	2
Never True	*Sometimes True*	*Always True*

7. I get nervous when I talk to new kids.

0	1	2
Never True	*Sometimes True*	*Always True*

8. I worry about what other children say about me.

0	1	2
Never True	*Sometimes True*	*Always True*

9. I only talk to kids that I know really well.

0	1	2
Never True	*Sometimes True*	*Always True*

10. I am afraid that other kids will not like me.

0	1	2
Never True	*Sometimes True*	*Always True*

_____Total Score, Social Anxiety Scale for Children

Interpreting Your Child's Score—A child's responses to any psychological test sometimes reflect concerns or feelings about very recent events, like what happened that day on the school bus, rather than ongoing problems. Because childhood social anxiety, even when pervasive, can also be temporary and can easily be confused with other anxieties and problems, a parent should not put great weight on a single test score. A high score does indicate, however, that further observation could be helpful. See chapter 17 for some considerations and tips on helping children cope with their social anxiety.

When interpreting your child's Social Anxiety Scale for Children score, keep in mind that girls tend to score higher than boys and that the scores of both sexes tend to decrease with age. Elementary school girls average a score of 10, with 70 percent of all girls scoring between 6 and 14. Boys average a score of 8, with 70 percent scoring between 4 and 12. By grade, scores tend to decrease from an average of 10 for children in the second and third grades to an average of 8 in the fifth and sixth grades. Although this scale has not been tested in older children, it is likely that social anxiety scores begin to increase with the new social stresses of adolescence.

15

BECOMING YOUR OWN THERAPIST

Welcome evermore to gods and men is the self-helping man. For him all doors are flung wide: him all tongues greet, all honors crown, all eyes follow with desire.

Ralph Waldo Emerson, 1841

Most people cope with their worst social fears in one of two ways: They fight them or they avoid them. Fighters look for opportunities to enter their feared situations. They take public speaking classes, approach people they fear, and hope that practice will lessen their anxiety. We admire their determination, and their efforts often succeed. Unfortunately, practice alone does not always make perfect when it comes to conquering social anxiety. When practice leads to the same old anxiety symptoms again and again, the results are dispiriting.

Avoiders try to cut their losses by opting out of their feared situations. They have found that discretion is the greater part of valor. These escape artists mange to hold anxiety at bay until the next time, but at a price of building their lives around avoiding embarrassment. They sacrifice some of the relatedness they want the most in order to avoid the anxiety that comes with being around people. But you can't avoid all of the people all of the time.

Either way, many people, having been unable to change, come to the erroneous conclusion that they *cannot* change. Depressed, some let their life aspirations fizzle out, or they rationalize that they never really wanted those social activities anyway. In fact, research has proven that people with social phobias can make changes and usually do change—when they use the right techniques.

In this chapter we outline a map for helping you find a way to manage and overcome social fears. Relief does not require that you spend years analyzing your childhood to try to figure out how you got this way. For most people with social anxiety who are willing to make a serious effort, learning some straightforward new approaches to deal with the problem can quickly lead to progress. Some people may find this program most useful as an adjunct to professional psychotherapy or medication treatments. Others may use this self-help program alone to help manage their social anxiety. We do not recommend this self-help program as a sole treatment for people with severe social phobia, or for people who have significant additional problems such as depression or alcoholism.

Our approach draws on techniques that have benefited people in our own clinical practices, in our research on treatment of social phobia, and in therapy research around the world. We have been particularly influenced by psychologist Richard Heimberg's pioneering work in group therapy of social phobia. The cognitive-behavioral principles that form the foundation for this approach are discussed in detail in chapter 10. Two guiding principles, however, bear special mention here.

THE STEP-BY-STEP APPROACH

It is paradoxical that while most people find it obvious that to walk from Point A to Point B you must take one step at a time, few are able to apply this principle to their persistent personal problems. With social anxiety problems, it is easy to get locked into an "all or none" way of thinking about change. In this mode of thinking, striving for anything less than perfection is not worth the effort, and achieving anything less than perfection is considered a failure. "Failures" mount and effort dissolves.

A step-by-step approach to overcoming social fears replaces big failures with a series of small successes. In our program, armed with new coping techniques, you will plan weekly forays into your feared social territory. Each of these exercises will challenge you with a slight increase in difficulty over the prior week's experiences. While the step-by-step approach may sound a bit slow-paced for problems you want solved yesterday, the time you will invest pales in comparison to the months and years too many people lose to the clutches of fear.

We are reminded of a doctoral student who had completed her courses, but who for years had been unable to start writing her final dissertation, which was expected to be about 150 pages in length. Like many a "professional" A.B.D. (all but dissertation), she was overwhelmed with anxiety over the enormity of her task. One of us (L.W.) recommended that she try to write no more than one page per day. Five months later she had completed her thesis, and within six months she had obtained her doctoral degree.

THE CONSTRUCTIVE APPROACH

Our program focuses on *constructing* a new set of coping skills (a positive goal), rather than a negative task of *eliminating* a fear. This constructive approach differs from conventional Western approaches to disorders or emotional problems. People with illnesses naturally hope for an effortless cure, like the penicillin that subdued deadly pneumonia in the 1940s. Some people with anxiety problems hope that the right therapist will simply reveal to them where they have gone wrong, or that a hypnotist will make the problems disappear. The focus on simple cures for difficult behavioral problems, however, is one reason why so many people fall short in their efforts at self-improvement, which often require the development of new skills.

The constructive approach begins with asking where you would like to be sometime in the future in terms of your social activities and abilities. Stating your goals in positive terms is the necessary first step toward achieving these goals.

Basic Ingredients

Three basic ingredients that need to be included in this formula for success are *productive thinking, exposure,* and *sustained motivation.*

Productive Thinking. It is a commonly accepted notion in psychology that highly negative thinking styles are associated with unpleasant emotional responses. If you enter a situation with fearful thoughts, such as "I'll never get through this speech," you will probably experience anxiety. If you focus on depressing thoughts like "No one cares about me," you are likely to feel depressed. Even when such negative thoughts are inaccurate (and they are often inaccurate in people with social anxiety), they can trigger or intensify negative emotions.

The good news about this connection is that if you work to neutralize the negative biases in the way you think about certain situations, you can affect your emotional state in a positive way. Change involves learning to identify negative thoughts that spring up automatically in certain situations—and learning to replace irrational or nonproductive thoughts with more rational and effective ones. "I will never get through this speech" becomes "I may feel uneasy at first, but it often gets better as I talk, and putting across my ideas to others will be satisfying."

Exposure. The behavioral principle for overcoming any fear or phobia is extraordinarily simple: Approach and do whatever you fear doing. To overcome a fear of driving, you need to approach and eventually drive the car. If your fear is public speaking, you must find audiences and speak to them.

Exposure therapy involves learning the methods that can make this principle work for you. This includes beginning with those situations you fear only mildly and building up to situations you fear the most. You may not want to begin working on your public speaking phobia by trying out a new stand-up comedy routine on *The Tonight Show.*

When therapeutic exposure is done properly, the tension that you experience at the beginning will dissipate as you "hang in there" and let your body naturally acclimate to the situation. The eventual drop in tension or anxiety is *reinforcing,* meaning it will make it easier for you to enter a fearful situation the next time it occurs.

Sustained Motivation. We are reminded of the old light bulb joke: How many psychoanalysts does it take to change a light bulb? Just one, but it must really want to change. By virtue of having read this far in the self-help chapter it seems likely that you have some "readiness" to embark on a program of change. But that's not enough either. It is one thing to get "psyched up" to begin a life change such as quitting smoking, losing weight, or organizing your professional life. It is quite another thing to *sustain* motivation when the change is sometimes painful in the short run and fully rewarding only down the road.

Motivation to change may falter in the face of anxiety and disappear when confronted with all-out fear. These are normal responses that you can anticipate and counteract by arranging immediate rewards (reinforcements) for hanging in. Better yet, the program you design can have reinforcements "built in." If simply following the program leads to its own rewards, there is no need to keep your eye on that elusive pot of gold at the end of the rainbow or to depend on another person to continuously cheerlead for you.

Following the step-by-step approach is also essential to keeping motivated. Each small success helps build the courage you need to reach for the next level. When you are ready to take on that challenge, the sense of accomplishment you will feel as you move to the next step is rewarding in itself.

Let's be realistic, though. Despite your best intentions and strong motivation, you are bound to encounter bumps on the road to success. It is important to acknowledge in advance that certain obstacles might trip you up and that events will not always go as planned. Lapses in progress or setbacks of this sort should not be cause for catastrophizing, but instead for regrouping and planning. Remember—*one lapse does not make a collapse!* Even a string of disappointments, or a "relapse," is not reason for abandoning your efforts, but instead signals the expected need for some more creative problem solving.

GETTING STARTED—PLANNING

Permanent behavior change requires some temporary schedule changes. To mount a successful self-change program you will need to arrange for time to implement it. Set aside at least one hour each week to complete your program tasks (three hours would be even better). If you find it difficult to allocate even one hour per week, then reconsider whether you should attempt the program at this time. Either your problems are too minor to deserve an hour per week of effort (possible), you are too busy with more important things than your mental health to invest an hour per week (unlikely), or you are experiencing some combination of fear about confronting your problems and skepticism about the effectiveness of our approach (very likely).

STEP 1: WHAT ARE YOUR GOALS?

Setting a goal sounds easy—after all, you know that you want to feel better. But translating that general desire into a useful goal is a crucial skill. Set your goals poorly—make them too lofty, too vague, unimportant to you, or impractical—and you surely will end up disappointed. On the other hand, well thought out goals will greatly increase your chances of success, and learning to set useful goals is a problem-solving skill you can use for the rest of your life.

You will need to formulate two types of goals. The first is the long-term goal. This is a statement about changes that you would like to achieve in, say, the next few months. The second type is the shorter-term "mini-goal"—the weekly goals that will help pave the way to accomplishing the larger overall goals. A young jazz musician with stage fright may wish to perform onstage with Wynton Marsalis one day, but his first step may be simply to get through next week's audition for his school band. To establish useful goals, it helps to follow some simple rules:

1. *Set goals for yourself, not for others.* You may hope that a certain person will find you more attractive if you become more socially assertive, but his or her behavior is not something you can directly control, so this would be a wasted goal. Instead set your sights on something you can do for yourself. A long-term goal to help maximize your appeal, for example, might be: ''I will take the initiative in getting to know Jeff better.''

2. *State long-term goals in positive terms.* Avoid setting goals for what you will *not* do, such as ''I will not stumble over any words when I speak.'' Instead ask yourself: What would I like to accomplish? ''I will speak up and discuss my ideas at staff meetings,'' and ''I will present a paper each year at the annual conference on ethics in accounting'' are goals stated positively.

3. *Goals should be behavioral, not emotional.* Avoid setting goals with reference to how you would like to feel, such as ''I will be totally at ease at parties.'' You cannot change your feelings directly. Instead, ask yourself what observable changes in your behavior would help you feel better about parties. The alternative statement, ''I will start up conversations with at least two people at each party,'' avoids mention of the need to feel a particular way. Improvement in the way you feel will *follow* achievement of your behavioral goals.

4. *Goal behaviors must be physically controllable.* Unless you are a master at yoga, replace goals for controlling involuntary symptoms such as sweating (''I won't sweat'') with goals about behavior you can potentially control (''I will maintain eye contact and continue the conversation even if I do sweat''). Improvement in uncontrollable symptoms such as sweating or trembling will occur as behavioral goals are achieved.

5. *Goals must be realistic.* While this may be difficult for you to judge at first, try to avoid goals that would seem grandiose even for an anxiety-free person (''I will give the greatest performance their ears have ever heard''). Such goals usually lead to disappointment. If you do happen to become the greatest thing since chopped liver, consider it icing on the cake!

6. *Goals must be clear and specific.* Avoid global statements such as "I will be more social." Exactly what does that mean? Will you have friends over for dinner parties? Will you attend socials or go to nightclubs? "Each month I will ask one friend to join me for dinner" is a clearly stated goal.

7. *Goals must be important to you.* Setting trivial or irrelevant goals will lead to diminishing interest and motivation. Don't be afraid to select the goals you have your heart set on.

The long-term goals you set become a sort of mission statement for your program. They serve as a guide for developing smaller weekly goals (mini-goals) as you proceed through a course of self-change. As you develop more effective coping responses and enter your feared situations more frequently, social anxiety will decrease. This reflects a basic tenet of behavioral psychology: How you feel (emotion) follows changes in what you do (behavior), rather than the other way around. Don't wait until it feels completely comfortable to get out and work toward your goals. The time is now!

Jill was a generally shy person when she began treatment. She was anxious dealing with people in most social activities and in her work at a bookstore. Rather than trying to change her whole personality, which she basically liked, she selected goals in a few areas of social behavior that she most wanted to change.

Jill's Overall Goals

1. I will initiate conversations with customers who approach my register.

2. I will accept invitations to some parties.

3. I will attend the Craft and Industry Fair; I will accept an invitation to perform a wool-spinning demonstration at the fair.

After Jill set these overall goals, she set a series of weekly mini-goals that included increasingly frequent and longer conversations with customers, accepting invitations to parties where close friends would be present, and attending crafts fairs but not performing spinning demonstrations quite yet. You will learn how to formulate mini-goals later on; but first, what are your overall goals? You may need to revise them a few times to be sure they meet the guidelines listed above.

What Are Your Overall Goals?

1. _____
   _____
   _____

2. _____
   _____
   _____

3. _____
   _____
   _____

A MAP TO GUIDE YOU— AN OVERVIEW OF THE PIC

The PIC (Personal Instruction Chart) is the organizing system for making step-by-step progress toward your overall social goals. The PIC helps you track your current achievements, breaks overall goals down into mini-goals and weekly tasks, and prompts you to organize your life so that accomplishing your goals is possible.

Each week, you will record current accomplishments, that week's social exposure goals (mini-goals), and strategy notes to help accomplish them. Once you have achieved the week's goals, you complete a new PIC: the past week's mini-goals become the current week's current accomplishments. The next step is then planned for the following week.

Insert copies of the blank PIC form into a notebook to allow you to keep a record of your progress. As you proceed through the program, accomplishing each week's mini-goals, turning each page will be a reminder that you are steadily accomplishing your overall mission.

Once you have established your long-term goal, what you would like to be able to accomplish after three months, it is time to plan the first step. Note that we do not ask you to plan the entire program up front. Adding too many instructions or steps all at once will eventually overwhelm almost anyone with anxiety. Don't bite off more than you can chew!

It is also impossible to plan your second step without seeing the results of the first step. Unexpected difficulties that crop up may need to be addressed. On the other hand, if the first step goes better than expected, you may want to aim a little higher next time.

The Personal Instruction Chart

Date:

Current Accomplishments	Weekly Mini-Goals

Strategy Notes (for reaching mini-goals)

STEP 2: CURRENT ACCOMPLISHMENTS

The next step is to write down what you have accomplished to date in the "Current Accomplishments" box. Say, for example, that your goal is to be able to give a talk in front of a large audience. Ask yourself what you can currently accomplish in the area of public presentations. Perhaps you already can present your ideas to a small group of colleagues (five or less). Or maybe you can put together the materials for a good presentation but cannot follow through with the presentation. In describing current accomplishments, you should follow some of the same rules you used for setting overall goals:

1. State your accomplishments in positive terms.
2. Accomplishments must be behavioral.
3. Accomplishments must be clear and specific.

You'll want to be even *more* specific here and in the mini-goals than you were in your overall goals. For planning purposes, it's not very helpful to write "I can give some speeches." Adding specifics such as "before a group of five or less" and "in an informal setting" provides the details you'll need to set future mini-goals. Your PIC might now look like the chart opposite:

STEP 3: WEEKLY MINI-GOALS

After you have recorded your current accomplishments, think about the next step in the direction of your overall goal. For many people, this will mean attempting activities you are currently avoiding. For example, if you can speak to five or fewer colleagues in an informal setting, the next mini-goal could be to give a presentation to five or fewer people in a *formal* setting, like a conference room or office (see page 158). Think of a specific presentation topic, place, and time for your goal.

If you are already able to attempt your feared activity (for example, give a speech), you may need to focus instead on improving the *quality* of your performance. This might involve setting mini-goals to increase your eye contact with the audience, to add a humorous story to a speech, or to improve your concentration on the content of your speech, rather than dwelling on distracting fears of the audience's criticism.

In devising your mini-goals, again refer back to the rules for overall goals. The only difference is that you need to *be as specific as possible*

Date: 7/1

Current Accomplishments	Weekly Mini-Goals
1. Can prepare speech 2. Can speak to 5 or fewer colleagues in an informal setting (e.g., at lunch)	

Strategy Notes (for reaching mini-goals)

in describing mini-goals. These should also be goals that you will have an opportunity to accomplish in the next week.

STEP 4: STRATEGY NOTES

To reach your week's goals, you will need to prepare some strategies. Under "Strategy Notes" you detail how you are going to get the job done. What specifically will you need to do to accomplish the mini-goal? It is not enough simply to say that you will do a, b, and c. It is important to "make arrangements" for accomplishing each goal.

Date: 7/1	

Current Accomplishments	**Weekly Mini-Goals**
1. Can prepare speech 2. Can speak to 5 or fewer colleagues in an informal setting (e.g., at lunch)	Speak to 5 or fewer colleagues about new sales ideas in conference room this week

Strategy Notes (for reaching mini-goals)

For example, if this week's task is to give a speech, it is critical that you plan when and where you will do this task (see opposite). You may also want to write down notes or even the full text of what you are going to say in your speech, as well as some helpful coping responses (see ''Core Techniques,'' page 161) that you might use during both practice sessions and the real thing.

Date: 7/1

Current Accomplishments

1. Can prepare speech
2. Can speak to 5 or fewer colleagues in an informal setting (e.g., at lunch)

Weekly Mini-Goals

Speak to 5 or fewer colleagues about new sales ideas in conference room this week

---

Strategy Notes (for reaching mini-goals)

1. Send E-mail invitations to 5 colleagues from sales department to meet on Tuesday 9 A.M. in conference room
2. Send copies of meeting agenda to same colleagues by Monday afternoon
3. Write notes for speech, practice giving speech daily
4. Develop a coping response and add it here:

STEP 5: GRADING YOUR EXERCISE

At the end of the social "exposure" (for example, after trying to give the speech), ask yourself, "Did I accomplish my mini-goal?" Note that this question is not "Did I accomplish my mini-goal without any anxiety?"

Avoid punishing yourself with "Yes . . . but" responses. Jill was making steady progress toward overcoming her fear and avoidance of talking with customers at the bookstore, but she had a tendency to

---

Date: 7/8

Current Accomplishments

1. I can talk to 5 or fewer colleagues in a formal setting (e.g., conference room)

Weekly Mini-Goals

1. Talk to 5–10 colleagues in conference room

Strategy Notes (for reaching mini-goals)

1. Prepare quarterly report to deliver to larger sales group
2. Send E-mail invitations to all 10 sales reps by Monday for Tuesday presentation
3. Remind myself daily of last week's success
4. Develop a coping response and add it here

---

belittle her accomplishments. After successfully completing an exposure task, she would catch herself saying "But it didn't count as progress because I was still a bit uptight." Eventually, Jill learned that changing her behavior was key and that her anxiety eventually diminished as she regularly practiced her new behaviors.

Review your PIC at the end of the week. If you succeeded in completing the mini-goals, fill out a new PIC. The past week's mini-goals become the next week's current accomplishments. Now you can devise new mini-goals and plan the next step with new strategy notes.

Filling out the next PIC symbolizes your success and tells you that you are inching closer to accomplishing your larger goals. Repeat this process each week until you achieve your overall goals.

If you are unable to achieve the mini-goals for a particular week, it is not a catastrophe or a reason to prematurely end your self-help program. In fact, if you were 100 percent successful in developing weekly tasks and accomplishing them, this would be quite extraordinary (and we might not believe it). There are several possible reasons for a slip. You might have set an overly-difficult or inappropriate mini-goal, in which case you should go back to that section of the PIC and develop an easier or more appropriate task. Or you might not have armed yourself with sufficient coping strategies and anti-anxiety tools. In this case, pick up the strategy notes section of your PIC with some of the suggestions made under the ''Core Techniques'' section below.

In summary, a key to success is to move one step at a time. Determine your goals by asking yourself what positive changes you would like to see. Start by reviewing your accomplishments to date and using them as a springboard for planning the next step, or mini-goal. Increase the likelihood that you will succeed by carefully planning strategy notes for accomplishing these goals. Finally, evaluate realistically how well you are doing, with an emphasis on praising yourself for making small steps toward accomplishing your goals.

CORE TECHNIQUES

PIC-UP I: Positive Coping Responses or, How to Get Your Head to Follow Your Body

Most people need more than just step-by-step exposure to their feared social activities in order to overcome their fears. As you design your first social exposure task you might well find yourself muttering ''I know I'll never get myself to do the speech in the first mini-goal, because I'll flip out first!'' This PIC-UP provides tools (or coping responses) that you can use on your journey through the PIC program.

The most important PIC-UP is a **positive coping response** you can make to yourself in a difficult social situation. As you may have guessed, focusing on images of yourself ''flipping out'' is *not* considered an effective coping response. It may, however, effectively work you into a frenzy. A more positive self-statement will serve to reduce overall fear and anxiety. Common examples include statements such as "I've done this before so I know I can do it," "I can't please everyone," and "I know I have a lot to say about this subject."

The coping responses that will work best for you should "speak" to your particular fearful thoughts. What types of negative thoughts do you typically carry with you into a feared social event? Learning to identify these **negative automatic thoughts (NATS)** is the first step toward generating a more productive way of thinking. NATS are pesky and not easily brushed aside. They are called **automatic** thoughts because they appear without effort—you've probably spent years "perfecting" these responses without knowing it. It won't take years to modify them, but it does require a systematic approach.

Record your negative thoughts on a PIC-UP I form, with columns for negative automatic thoughts and coping responses.

PIC-UP I: NATS

Negative Automatic Thoughts	Coping Responses
1. They will think I am stupid	
2. I will never get through this meeting	
3. I have nothing worthwhile to say	
4.	
5.	

Some people say they can't recall having any NATS about their feared situation. Almost invariably, the negative thoughts are there but have become so automatic that they hardly register. If you can't recall any NATS, make a point of jotting down your fearful thoughts *immediately* following a stressful social event.

Listed below are some categories of garden-variety NATS that typify the thinking errors of socially anxious people. Categorizing each NAT before you begin the task of changing it is a helpful exercise, because it will increase your awareness of the types of errors that are part of your thinking style. Do you overgeneralize, practice mind reading, or turn predictions into facts? We recommend that you categorize each of your NATS in the beginning of your program, so that you can get used to looking for similar types of thinking errors in the future. After you get the hang of this, you can move directly from NATS to the next step (challenging them), without categorizing the NATS.

Common Species of NATS
(A.K.A. Cognitive Distortions)

1. *Perfectionism.* "If my speech isn't as good as the best I've ever heard, I will have failed." By setting an impossible goal, you set yourself up for failure.

2. *Prospecting for Flaws.* "If I see one person in the audience frown, I'll be very disappointed" (even if fifty other people are nodding and smiling). You pick out a small flaw and dwell on it alone, ignoring any positive experiences.

3. *Discounting the Positive.* "I had a good time at the last few parties, but that was pure luck. This party will be a disaster." You dismiss positive experiences as if they don't count. In this way you prevent yourself from learning from good experiences.

4. *Turning Predictions into Facts.* "I know I won't be able to think of anything to say." You predict things will turn out bad, and you treat your prediction like an established fact.

5. *"Should" Statements.* "I should always be relaxed with people." With "should" statements you judge and punish yourself, without dealing with the problem itself.

6. *Mind Reading.* "He'll think I'm pathetic if he sees my hand tremble." You assume that someone will react negatively to

you, and you never bother to check out whether your assumption was correct.

7. *All-or-None Thinking.* "My whole performance will be a wasted effort unless everyone likes it." You view your performance in black and white terms, leaving no room for doing merely an excellent job.

8. *False Theory of Relativity.* "She is always completely at ease. I'll look terrible relative to her." You build up others to an unrealistic extent at the same time you tear yourself down.

9. *Overgeneralization.* "She didn't want to go out with me— nobody will ever want to go out with me." You see a single negative event as a never-ending pattern.

10. *Emotional Reasoning.* "I feel insecure, so everyone must see me as a failure." You assume that the way you feel is the objective reality.

11. *Assuming the Center of the Universe.* "My boss is so critical— he must hate me." You take it personally and ignore the fact that your boss is critical of everybody.

Challenging the Common NAT. After you have decided the types of errors you are making (most people make many types), the next step is to challenge each of the negative and usually irrational thoughts by asking yourself a series of questions:

"Am I one hundred percent sure that my NAT is true?"

"Have I *ever* been successful in this type of situation?"

"Is it at all possible that some other result will occur . . . something other than what I fear will happen?"

"What is the worst that can happen?"

"What are the *real odds* that my feared idea will happen?"

"What would an objective friend or outsider predict will happen instead of what I think will happen?"

The goal here is to generate a more productive way of viewing the situation, one that will be more rational and will lead to less of an emotionally charged response.

Let's pursue the common NAT "They will think that I am stupid" (an example of "mind reading"). Are you 100 percent sure that you will be viewed as stupid? Will absolutely everyone think that what you have to say is stupid? Have you ever been in a similar situation and had people think that you were not stupid (did some observers even think the opposite)? Use the answers to these questions to construct a more positive coping response, and record this summary statement on the PIC-UP I (see page 166).:

If you are having trouble developing a coping response, go back to reviewing your NATS. If they are too general or vague, you may need to make them more specific. For example, take a too-vague general NAT, "I'm a mess," and carry it through to its illogical conclusion: "I'm a mess because . . . I fear my hands will tremble . . . and everyone will notice . . . and they'll think I'm a drug addict . . . and soon I'll have no friends and no career!" Now we have some more juicy specific fears that we can question in order to develop more useful coping responses.

Think through what an upcoming feared situation will be like *before* you jump in. Imagine what types of nonproductive thoughts will tend to spring up automatically and record these NATS. People tend to treat their NATS as if they were facts; instead, think of them as untested hypotheses. While facts are indisputable, hypotheses are educated guesses that can be tested to determine their truthfulness. Now you can generate a more realistic idea and record this under "Coping Responses" in the PIC-UP I.

It is crucial to develop a coping response statement that you can believe in, rather than mouthing a phony slogan. If the response doesn't feel right, go back to challenging the NAT until you come up with a more credible alternative. For example, Jim was struggling with anxiety about an upcoming speech to his fellow salespeople, when his massage therapist recommended that he use the "affirmation" that she always found helpful: "I know that I will act in a professional and competent way." Jim tried it out for size, but found that it just didn't seem to speak directly to his own fear that people would be bored by his talk. After grilling himself with the type of questions mentioned earlier, Jim came up with the coping statement "I know I have some good ideas, and people have told me so." He knew this was true, and he found that he experienced tension relief just by uttering the phrase.

Building a Coping Response into Your Strategy. When you plan a weekly mini-goal, record a coping response in the "Strategy Notes" section of the original PIC.

Build the coping response into your practice sessions. On the day of the planned social exposure (such as the presentation to five colleagues from the sales department mentioned in the PIC), say the new

Negative Automatic Thoughts	Coping Responses
1. They will think I am stupid 2. I will never get through this meeting 3. I have nothing worthwhile to say 4. 5.	1. I am actually reasonably intelligent 2. I've gotten through these meetings before. There is no reason I can't do it again! 3. I have some good ideas

coping response to yourself silently before the meeting as well as during your presentation. Remember that the coping response embodies the whole rational approach you have worked on during the week.

PIC-UP II: Think Exposure

The key to improvement is confronting the social situations or events you fear. Every time you avoid or escape feared situations, you experience immediate but fleeting relief of anxiety. Despite its long-term drawbacks, this drop in tension or anxiety is extremely

Date: 7/8

Current Accomplishments	Weekly Mini-Goals
1. Can prepare speech 2. Can speak to 5 or fewer colleagues in an informal setting (e.g., at lunch)	1. Speak to 5 or fewer colleagues about new sales ideas in conference room this week

Strategy Notes (for reaching mini-goals)

1. Send E-mail invitations to 5 colleagues from sales department to meet on Tuesday 9 A.M. in conference room
2. Send copies of meeting agenda to some colleagues by Monday afternoon
3. Write notes for speech, practice giving speech daily
4. Coping response: "I have some good ideas"
5. Review NATS and coping responses each day before and after practicing.

rewarding, thereby increasing the likelihood that you will avoid similar situations in the future. The more you are able to let yourself move in the other direction, even going to extremes in exposing yourself to feared situations, the more rapidly you will progress.

Welcome this period of self-directed change as an opportunity to experiment with new social behaviors and situations. Plan events that take you a bit beyond your usual style or habits. Make conversation with the cashier at the grocery story if you typically remain quiet, or ask a group of strangers for directions even if you don't really need them.

Push yourself to try these new behaviors on for size during this experimental phase of your life. Remember, you have little to lose in such practice encounters, even if your worst fears were to come to pass. When the practice goes well, you'll be able to transfer some of your new confidence to dealing with the situations that bother you most.

If you feel unsure of yourself in these kinds of situations, think of people you know who are good at them. How would they handle these events? What would they say? How would they speak? Do not try to "become" one of these people, but select one or two specific aspects of their social behaviors as a model for your own behavior. Jill, for example, was having trouble thinking of things to say to customers at the bookstore. She decided to pay more attention to her coworker Kate, who always seemed to be having a great time with customers. Kate sometimes started a conversation by saying something positive about the book a customer was buying. Jill tried this out and discovered that it worked well for her as a natural conversation starter.

PIC-UP III: The Assertive Option

Shy people often deal with their fears of confrontation by holding back their thoughts or feelings. They overestimate the danger of speaking up and seek protection in their silence. This may allow for a temporary sense of safety, but at a price. Common consequences of not speaking up are anger directed toward oneself ("How can I be such a wimp and let him run over me again!") or toward the more outspoken person ("How could he be so insensitive to my feelings?"). But when you don't allow your voice to be heard, is it reasonable to expect others to be able to read your mind? The outspoken person may interpret the bashful person's silence in a number of ways: He or she may assume that the silent person is not interested, is angry, is silently thinking badly of him or her, or is silently agreeing with him or her.

Silence and avoidance are strategies you might occasionally use to handle difficult situations. But is having avoidance as your only option worth the price for you? Does it produce positive results? Another choice is the **assertive option.** This involves telling a person exactly what you want in a calm way that does not antagonize. The assertive option is simple in form and is usually well received by others, even if they disagree with what you have to say. In most situations, other people respond positively when they are given news in an honest, straightforward manner that shows respect for their own feelings or attitudes. In cases where others *do mind* hearing a point of view other than their own, a simple coping response spoken silently, such as "I have the right to present my own views" (see PIC-UP I) can bolster your confidence. You can implement the assertive option in four steps:

First Step: **Acknowledge** the other person's point of view by saying something positive (for example, when talking to a boss: "I understand what you are saying about the costs of changing our record keeping. You make a good point").

Second Step: **Assert** your own agenda by saying what you want or what you are thinking ("I believe we should change the way we keep financial records because the costs will actually be lower in the long run").

Third Step: **Stay calm** no matter what response you receive from the other person (for example, your boss is screaming "All I care about is this month's balance sheet," but you are nodding while rehearsing a PIC-UP I to yourself: "Even if he screams now, after he calms down he'll respect me for having spoken up").

Fourth Step: **Cycle back** to the first step if the other person does not seem to hear or understand your thought (return to saying "I understand your point, but I wanted you to know my thoughts about it because you asked me to do the analysis").

You have the right to be heard as long as you put forth your message in a way that is not hurtful to other people. The assertive option provides a path for making your voice heard in a nonthreatening way.

PIC-UP IV: Role Playing

Musician to passerby: "How do I get to Carnegie Hall?"
Passerby: "Practice, practice, practice."

Old joke of unknown origin

Social behavior is a skill much like any other, such as playing the piano or tying your shoes. The importance of practice cannot be overemphasized. The difference is that while you can practice tying your shoes however and whenever you like, social situations are less controllable, so that arranging the practice of social skills can be challenging. You can overcome this obstacle, however, if you have a friend or family member who is willing to role-play feared social events with you. Your partner can play the role of job interviewer, potential date, audience member for a speech or a wedding toast, and so on.

Even though it may seem odd at first, you should make role plays as realistic as possible. If you are going to simulate giving a toast, take out a wineglass and hold it in the air while you speak. For a job interview role play, arrange your chairs as they might be placed during the real-life interview. Ask your partner to stay "in role" (no kidding around) for as long as it takes to approximate a sample of the real thing.

Ask your partner to avoid being too easy on you. When Rick wanted to practice negotiating a sales agreement with a client, he asked his friend to drive a moderately hard bargain and not to give in too easily. Afterward, ask your partner for honest but constructive feedback. The emphasis should be on what you did well and how you might improve upon your performance, rather than on destructive criticism about what you did "wrong."

Just prior to beginning a role play, generate one or two coping responses that you can state to yourself during the exercise. For example, if you fear that other people will think a speech is boring, you may want to remind yourself, "Some people have told me they find my ideas interesting" during a pause in your presentation. As mentioned in PIC-UP I, a productive cognitive coping phrase reduces anxiety, whereas self-critical thoughts increase anxiety.

Also, set a reasonable goal before you begin. Don't be embarrassed to set a particular goal because it seems too easy, such as "Just complete the role play" or "Use my assertive option." Monitor your anxiety by writing down your anxiety level using a 0 to 10 scale (where 0 represents no anxiety and 10 represents the most severe anxiety possible) every minute or so. After completing the role play, first decide whether you accomplished your goal: yes or no. Second, examine your pattern of anxiety scores. Were you most anxious at the beginning of the role play? At the end? Note any connections between your anxiety scores and any negative thoughts you were entertaining at those moments. If you started out by thinking "She will think I'm an idiot!" you would probably notice higher anxiety scores associated with that thought. Use this practice time to "get cognitive" with yourself: Think about what specific negative thoughts you experienced, challenge their truthfulness, and replace them with more productive statements about yourself and the situation. Then try the role play again.

When the "wrong" guy was pressing Claudia for a date, she felt guilty about turning him down, fearing that he would get upset or feel bad. Despite knowing deep down that it would be best for both of them in the long run if she said no, she lacked confidence that she would be able to stand up to this guy's persistence. She enlisted the help of her roommate's boyfriend, Carlos, to role-play a scene in which she successfully used her assertive skills to turn down the date. She asked Carlos to purposely play out a worst-case scenario. Part of it went something like this:

CARLOS: So, Claudia, how about coming to a movie with me tonight?

CLAUDIA: Sorry, but I have some other plans.

CARLOS: But you always seem to have other plans. Are you going out with somebody?

CLAUDIA: I'm flattered that you're so persistent, but I just don't think it would work out for us to date.

CARLOS: C'mon, Claudia, you're not being fair if you don't even give me a chance.

CLAUDIA: I don't want to hurt your feelings, and I'd like to be friends, but you make me uncomfortable when you don't hear what I'm saying.

CARLOS: What do you mean I don't hear? I hear you saying "Get lost!"

CLAUDIA: Carlos, that's not what I'm saying, but if you can't talk without yelling, I'm afraid I have to go now.

Claudia was surprised by how real the exercise felt. It helped that Carlos really got into it when he was playacting the "wrong guy" and didn't give up easily. Claudia found that while she was somewhat anxious during the role play, she was able to hang in there and accomplish her goal of using her assertive option. The coping phrase "I don't owe him an explanation for why I won't go out with him" was helpful, and she felt empowered at the end of the role play. In real life, the guy got the message more quickly—and without the yelling or extreme hurt feelings that Claudia had originally feared.

PIC-UP V: Relaxation

Some people find it helpful to slow down their engines just prior to entering an anxiety-producing situation. Actors, for example, will commonly use some form of relaxation exercise moments before the curtain rises. There are many ways to achieve a relaxed state, including self-hypnosis, meditation, yoga, and breathing control exercises, to name but a few. A method called deep muscle relaxation is particularly helpful in calming the body's fight-or-flight system, which is responsible for many symptoms of anxiety.

Deep muscle relaxation involves first tensing particular muscle groups, then "letting them go" or relaxing those same muscle groups. After finding a comfortable and quiet spot to sit or lie down, begin "at the bottom" by tightening up your toes. Hold them tight for 10 to 15 seconds, and then relax them for 10 to 15 seconds. Say the words "Let them go" as you relax the muscles. Repeat the process with each of the following muscle groups: calves, thighs, buttocks, stomach, shoulders, neck (forward), neck (backward), face, forearms, and fists. As you are releasing each of these muscle groups, think of your body as becoming totally relaxed and heavy, sinking into your chair or couch. Once you have finished with all the muscles, allow yourself to lie quietly for a few minutes. If you notice any residual tension in any of the muscle groups, then once again tense them and let them go.

Deep muscle relaxation works best if you start by trying it in situations where you are not extremely anxious. It may take some practice, so it is best to devote ten or fifteen minutes to it daily. Once you find it working, try to gradually add it to your cognitive methods for dealing with anxiety over upcoming situations. Attacking social anxiety in your body as well as in your mind can improve your control over it.

TROUBLESHOOTING GUIDE

We've given you a lot of ideas on how to move forward and overcome your social fears, but what if certain things go wrong? The guide below can help you put it all together.

What If . . .

A. I can't make my goals behavioral
B. I seem not to have any NATS
C. I can't think of any mini-goals
D. I can't successfully challenge my NATS
E. I can't really believe my positive coping response
F. I'm afraid to do my planned exposure
G. I succeed at my first mini-goals, but then it gets harder
H. My feared situations rarely occur in real life; how can I practice them?

I. My new assertiveness is a problem; someone doesn't like it
J. My anxiety seems physical; I can't stop blushing
K. I have a supercritical boss whom *everyone* fears; it's not just me!
L. I can't get motivated to work on this

. . . Then Try This

A. I can't make my goals behavioral. Think about what differences *others* might notice in you once you have improved. Or imagine that someone else was observing you with a hidden videocamera as you improved. What would these people see that is different about you? Would you go somewhere you've avoided going, say something you've avoided saying, change your physical behavior (for example, make more eye contact)?

If you are one of the relatively few people with social anxiety who actually does not avoid any physical behaviors, take a look at your cognitive "behaviors." Jane, for example, was giving frequent speeches and receiving compliments for her fine work. She wasn't avoiding any behaviors, but her thoughts during the speeches strayed to terror that others would notice her blushing and trembling. Jane set a goal of keeping her attention on the subject of her speech, rather than allowing herself to dwell on her anxiety symptoms.

B. I seem not to have any NATS. At first, try looking for these automatic thoughts *as they occur* when you are anxious. Write them down as soon as possible. If that does not work, ask yourself the general question "What do I seem to fear in this situation?" Do not worry that it may not be identical to your precise thoughts. This will give you an approximate cognition to work with. Some people suppress their NATS, disturbed that they seem too embarrassing or foolish—but that's the point! Get them out and observe their senselessness in the light of day.

C. I can't think of any mini-goals. Once you have determined your overall goal ("I want to be able to make sales presentations to the boards of other companies") and you have listed your current accomplishments ("I can make small presentations to two or three familiar people without getting anxious"), ask yourself what the *next smallest improvement* would be (for example, making presentations to two or three people where one of the persons is a stranger). Some people reject such potential mini-goals, believing that a small change is not worthy of an effort. Don't let yourself use this all-or-none thinking as an excuse to avoid taking the first step toward change.

D. I can't successfully challenge my NATS. Think of yourself as an attorney cross-examining a witness. In this case, the attorney has the attitude you would like to develop and the witness has your irrational fears. Demand answers from yourself to tough questions: "Mr. Worry-wart, what evidence do you have that no one will appreciate your ideas? Are you absolutely positive that everyone present will be horrified that you spoke up?" Alternatively, put yourself in the shoes of your audience. What do you notice about a speaker when you're in the audience? When you hear a speaker stumble, do you conclude that he or she is stupid?

E. I can't really believe my positive coping response. You may not have sufficiently convinced yourself of the flaws in your irrational thoughts. Return to challenging your NATS and use the suggestions above. Develop a coping response that speaks directly to your fears.

F. I'm afraid to do my planned exposure. Practice using a cognitive coping response (see above) as you imagine doing your exposure. Remind yourself that you are doing "experiments in living" right now in order to improve your social skills. This will help you separate yourself a bit from the situation and develop a more productive perspective. If you are still stuck, you have probably set too ambitious a goal and need to scale it back and try again.

G. I succeed at my first mini-goals, but then it gets harder. You have become accustomed to avoiding or escaping these situations. It is only natural that you become anxious when the situations become more difficult. Review your progress to date and remind yourself of your accomplishments. Be sure you haven't set too large a step for yourself. You may want to practice situations at the level of your previous step until you are more completely comfortable with moving on. As you move higher, you may need to put some extra effort into challenging NATS.

H. My feared situations rarely occur in real life; how can I practice them? Events such as giving a toast at a wedding or appearing on the *Today* show to promote a book do not occur very often. Finding a friend, spouse, or group of friends who will help you practice (role-play) the event is of tremendous help in such cases. Role playing can be awkward for some adults who haven't played imaginary characters since childhood. Do yourself a favor and try it anyway.

I. My new assertiveness is a problem; someone doesn't like it. You cannot please everybody. When done correctly, assertive behavior is usually effective, but a few people may wish you were still a pushover. Remember this when you are using your assertive option so that you can put disappointing events into perspective: "I did my best to respect his position *and* tell him what I want. . . . I guess I can't please everyone all of the time.''

J. My anxiety seems physical; I can't stop blushing. The best approach is not to try to eliminate all blushing (or sweating or palpitations). This is a setup for failure. Instead, put blushing in perspective: ''So what if I blush? It just means the blood vessels in my cheeks like to show off.'' Try announcing to friends that you blush a lot and see how they react to it. Ask them to try to make you blush so you can practice your coping response. When you are able to use such cognitive coping strategies (challenging your fears about the terrible consequences of blushing), you will actually blush less, simply because you will be less self-conscious.

K. I have a supercritical boss whom *everyone* fears; it's not just me! All your fears may not be irrational. (In psychology we have a saying—''Even paranoid people have real enemies.'') But you still need to develop adequate coping strategies to deal with your response to such a person. If this boss is mean to everyone, why are you taking it personally? How do others deal with him? Use these questions to help yourself develop positive coping responses.

L. I can't get motivated to work on this. If you can't get motivated, reassess how much you want to change and whether fear is holding you back. Deciding *not* to change is a choice, just as deciding *to* change is a choice. When viewed this way, your task is to decide which particular choice would be best for you. Will your life improve if you overcome your social fears? Is it worth putting some effort into change? No one can decide this but you. If you do want to change but remain blocked by fear, working with a mental health professional can help you get started.

BUILDING SOCIAL SKILLS

In addition to using the PIC to manage anxiety, some people will benefit from learning specific social skills to use in particular situations. While a complete treatment of this subject is beyond the scope of this book, we have included a few additional ideas if you're thinking about . . .

Dating

One of the biggest mistakes people of both sexes make is thinking that each date should lead to an ultimate love mate. This is a classic all-or-none thinking error. It creates excessive pressure and sets you up for disappointment. An alternative view is that the date can be an opportunity to get out and have a nice time. Pick activities that you would personally enjoy and focus on fun rather than love.

If a date does not go well, try not to be such a tough critic of your own performance. Research on dating suggests that a key to ultimate success is to keep up your frequency of efforts. In other words, the best way to become good at dating is to go on a lot of dates. Think of each date as another opportunity to practice your dating skills.

For those who have been out of practice for a while, seek out advice from people who are good at dating. A person of the opposite sex can be a particularly good source of information. It may be useful for a man to ask a close woman friend if she would help him shop for new clothes. Friends or coworkers might be helpful in recommending some good first date activities they have enjoyed.

On the first date, you may be nervous about thinking of what to say or talk about. Lean on "open-ended" questions that often lead to interesting conversations, such as "What do you do in your spare time?" or "What's your job like?" as opposed to "Yes-No" questions, which can be conversation killers. Asking open-ended questions shows that you are interested in your date and allows the other person to share the conversation without feeling burdened.

And listen to the answers! Some people are so preoccupied with thinking of what to say next, or with the impression they are making, that they don't pay attention to the answers their date is giving. In that answer is the material that will allow the conversation to continue naturally.

If you have had a nice time once the date is over (remember, your goal is just to have a pleasant time), then say so. People like to hear this when it is said directly and simply. That way, there is less guessing about who felt what. Remember, the other person may have the same worries and anxieties about the date as you do. Finally, whether you are a man or a woman, if you would like to see the person again, take the initiative to call the next day and ask for a second date. The person will usually be pleased that you asked. The worst that can happen is that he or she will say no. Remember, most dating relationships end soon after they have started, and it is usually not possible to determine the reason afterward.

Public Speaking

Be prepared.

Old Boy Scout Honor Pledge

Think of a speech as an opportunity to communicate ideas, rather than as a test of your public speaking skills. Audiences are generally much more interested in what you have to say than in the particulars of how you say it.

In some cases, anxiety about an upcoming speech or presentation leads people to avoid careful preparation. Just thinking about preparing may lead to thoughts and images of a disastrous attempt. If you know your stuff well, you will better be able to confront negative cognitions such as "I won't know what to say." Try reading your speech or reciting your comments for a meeting into a tape recorder. It is actually not so important to listen to the tape; just practicing with the tape recorder helps get people used to speaking aloud in front of an audience. When you are ready, ask a friend or two to serve as an audience and recite the speech to them. Follow the procedures discussed earlier under "PIC-UP IV: Role Playing."

Study the speaking habits of excellent public speakers, including those you might see on television. Pick out one or two things they do that you find appealing. When one of us took a moment to pay attention to the particular public speaking habits of a well-known psychiatrist, some of the speaker's techniques became evident. He would dramatically increase the intensity and volume of his voice when making an important point and would respond to audience questions by moving toward the questioner and making eye contact as he spoke.

Attending Parties with Strangers

Almost everyone can relate to feeling nervous about going to a party at some time in their lives. If you don't know most of the people at the party, the coping phrase "Who cares if they like me or not" is often helpful. After all, if you they don't know you and you may never see them again, why not cash in the chips and go for broke? Again, as with dating and public speaking, it is useful to focus on the opportunity to communicate and meet some people, rather than to view the party as an examination.

From a behavioral point of view, try "jumping in" to a conversation as soon as you arrive at a party. If the first or second try does not work out very well, then jump in with yet another group of people and let your presence be known. Most strangers do not end up hitting it off and becoming best friends. The more conversations you enter, the greater the likelihood that eventually you will find a group of people you enjoy. Remember to use open-ended questions such as "What are you guys talking about?" or "What do you think about this party?" Traditional (and seemingly corny) entrées can also do the job of ice-breaking: "Mind if I join in?" "Come here often?" or occasionally even "Have I seen you somewhere before?"—but probably not "What's a nice person like you . . ."

If conversation doesn't come easily to you, arm yourself with a story about yourself or a joke that might be appropriate to tell if the opportunity comes up. Total spontaneity is nice, but don't let yourself get caught up in an all-or-none thinking about this situation too. A little planning can lessen anxiety, and ultimately this will allow you to be more spontaneous.

AFTER SUCCESS

When you have accomplished your goal, don't throw this chapter away. Social anxiety problems are not one-shot deals; they're not like a case of the measles that grants you lifetime immunity. Wherever your life is heading, social anxieties may come with the territory. The difference is that now you will have the know-how to manage any flare-up before it becomes a big problem.

Jill, for example, admits that while she routinely chats with customers at the store, every once in a while she starts dwelling on negative thoughts about her performance and gets some tinges of nervousness. Instead of becoming overwhelmed and clamming up, as she used to, she pulls out the cognitive-behavioral techniques she has learned to manage social anxiety. For a small lapse, she might try to identify what unwanted thoughts are entering her consciousness and challenge their unrealistic qualities. If the problem continues to bother her for a few days, she pulls out the PIC and begins to record "where she's at," designs mini-goals, and brainstorms strategies for moving forward again.

After her divorce at age twenty-eight, Jennifer found many of her old social fears resurfacing, despite all of the gains she had made a few years ago in therapy for phobia of public speaking. Now that she was on her own again, she found that going alone to public events and parties was surprisingly anxiety provoking. Fortunately, when it came to dealing with her anxiety, she was not starting from scratch. Once Jennifer recognized that her social anxiety was just a variation on an old theme, she knew she could deal with it. She had a lot of recently acquired coping skills buried somewhere in her social repertoire. When she systematically applied these skills to her new problems, she progressed much faster than she had the first time she had tackled her social anxiety. Anxiety will come and go, but coping skills can be available to you for life.

Finally, if you find it too difficult to make headway with a self-help approach, you needn't feel all is lost. Enlisting the help of a "guide" in the form of a therapist can provide the extra push you may require. For many people, the added reinforcement delivered by an objective outside expert who reviews your work, contributes ideas for weekly goals and coping tips, and cheers your accomplishments with you can mean the difference between disappointment and success.

16

SELF-HELP VIGNETTES

*You gain strength, courage, and confidence by every experience
in which you really stop to look fear in the face.*

Eleanor Roosevelt

CHLOE'S STORY:
"I'M NOT GOING TO TAKE IT ANYMORE!"

It was on Chloe's thirtieth birthday that she decided enough was
enough. While her secretarial job in the city was okay, she felt that
her life was drifting by without the career she wanted. Growing up
in a working-class family with four younger brothers, Chloe had always longed to be in a profession that involved helping children. She
knew that a college education would be the key to opening up her
options in this area. In the past, however, thinking about her goal was
as far as Chloe had progressed toward it.

Chloe's problem was not that she lacked the money, drive, or intelligence needed for college. She had received good grades in high school
and her guidance counselor had urged her to apply. Chloe had refused.
At the time, she had rationalized her decision to take a secretarial job,
telling herself that she would be happier earning good money right
away. The real reason was her fear of speaking up in a classroom.

In high school, she would never volunteer an answer to a question
or contribute to a class discussion, although there was much she
wanted to say. She would nervously prepare for class presentations

assigned by her teacher, only to cave in to her public speaking fears and feign being sick on her day to speak. Her teachers and family made the mistake of accommodating her avoidance. Teachers liked Chloe, and they would go easy on her lack of participation while giving her credit for her solid written work. Her parents were very traditional and never placed much emphasis on their daughter's school achievement. She could become a happy wife and mother, they thought, without giving speeches. Now Chloe used her thirtieth birthday as a starting point for the change she had long wanted.

Chloe responded to an ad in a local newspaper about a treatment study at the medical center on public speaking fears. Because she was unable to travel across town for the weekly appointments the research program required, Chloe was offered a referral to another clinic or a self-help version of a treatment program. She chose the latter and followed the steps of a self-help manual while making only monthly visits to one of us (L.W.) in order to review her progress.

In the beginning, Chloe worked on developing several clear and objective goals. The task was not as easy as it seemed, because she realized that she had only vague ideas of her ultimate goals, including going to college and working with children. Following the instructions of the self-help manual, Chloe tried to be more specific: "What exactly will I need and want to accomplish in the area of my public speaking fear in order to achieve my career goals?" She decided that the first major step was definitely college, and to succeed in college she would need to be able to speak up in class. She decided to set an overall goal for the therapy of being able to speak up in front of others when she had something to say.

With this overall goal in mind, Chloe began to think about shorter-term tasks that "placed end to end" would ultimately accomplish the bigger goal. This was not simple either, because she had arranged her current life so that she didn't have to do any public speaking. She would need to create some opportunities to do public speaking in order to expose herself to her feared situation.

She remembered that she had recently declined a request from her church to give a talk about her experience as a volunteer in a local Big Brother–Big Sister program. This could be one intermediate step, but it still seemed too much to try all at once. After all, her current accomplishments in public speaking were limited to telling a story to two, or at most three, people, and never a formal speech. Chloe decided that her first mini-goal would be to simply tape-record a formal speech about her volunteer experience. This was no small step, considering that she disliked the sound of her voice and even hated leaving messages on answering machines.

Chloe used the speech not only to talk about her experience, but also to organize her personal views on how society neglects its children. She began to get into it and even found herself looking forward to making the recording. To deal with her fears of sounding "bad" to others, she developed a coping response to say to herself during the talk, reminding herself that her goal was "to provide information to people" rather than to be judged.

At first she performed her talk in front of a mirror and with the tape recorder—her anxiety level was surprisingly low. Next she got up the nerve to tell a couple of friends about her project, and they enthusiastically agreed to serve as a practice audience. As she proceeded with her speech, she noticed feeling short of breath. She reminded herself to keep her focus on telling her story, and the feeling passed. Afterward, she asked for some feedback, and her friends reported that they had found the talk to be very interesting, but that she should slow down so they could better follow her ideas.

Chloe realized she had gotten short of breath because she had been racing to get her talk over with. She incorporated the advice of her friends into new coping responses: "People will appreciate it if I take my time" and "I have something interesting to communicate." In her next talk, given in front of a few friends, she tried pausing after a key point and filling the pause with her silent coping responses. In this way she naturally slowed down and gave her confidence a boost as well.

Her next goal was to give the same talk in front of a small group at her church. Chloe was more nervous because it was a larger group, but she was also more confident because of her recent good experiences. Again the talk went well, and Chloe tried to bring her newfound speaking confidence into her everyday activities, setting mini-goals to push herself to speak up at a meeting at work and wherever else she could.

Gradually Chloe began to feel that she had the capacity to participate in a college classroom. Because she still felt apprehensive about college, though, she continued to use the self-help program to help her get through the process of calling admissions offices and getting through interviews. She planned out her week's goal by writing it down on her self-help record sheet, along with notes about when and whom to call. After accomplishing a goal, she would immediately write down goals for the following week, to keep her next step in mind.

Chloe managed to enroll in her first class well before her thirty-first birthday. While she remained somewhat nervous about the possibility of giving class presentations, she was now determined to go through with them anyhow. She ended her monthly therapy visits.

In a follow-up session six months later, Chloe reported that she was still advancing through both school and her fears. She had experienced a minor setback two months earlier, reacting badly to another student's criticism of her comments in class. Fearing an anxiety relapse and alarmed to find herself even considering a retreat back to full-time secretarial life, Chloe pulled out her self-help manual, reminded herself that one slip didn't mean she was finished, and began setting small weekly goals once again. She returned to making speeches in front of some friends, but this time asked them to challenge her with critical remarks and tough questions. After toughening herself up a bit in this way, Chloe was back on track toward her goals.

A CURE FOR A PRAYER

Every once in a while we hear a story of a person who has overcome a social anxiety problem completely on his or her own. Ethan, a successful thirty-five-year-old corporate vice president, was bewildered by his particular fear. In accord with his family's religious practices, Ethan recited a brief prayer each Friday night after his wife lit the Jewish Sabbath candles. Ethan, who would frequently make high-level presentations to his company's board of directors or give public presentations on economic matters, was surprised to find himself becoming extremely anxious about properly delivering the Friday night prayer. Why, he thought, should he become anxious in the company of his wife, his wife's parents, and his own three children?

After much reflection, Ethan concluded that his fear could be explained by the high expectations he placed on himself in this particular situation. He knew that his family members held him in high esteem: He was a successful breadwinner as well as a beloved father and spouse. But he also knew that he was very human. He worried that his family members would notice some fault . . . a chink in the armor that would lead them to lose confidence in him.

Following this insight, Ethan decided to disclose his fear to his family one Friday evening before the prayer: "I would like to ask you all something that may sound silly, but which is very important to me. . . . I sometimes worry that I will let you all down in some way. That you might notice that I'm only human . . ." The response from his family was overwhelming. One by one they approached him with a big hug. His fourteen-year-old son summed up their sentiment: "We've always known you're only human, Dad. We love you anyway!"

Ethan reported that after that evening he never again became nervous while reciting the prayer: "I recall my son's words and I feel at ease." Without reading any self-help manuals, Ethan had identified a negative automatic thought that seemed to be the source of his anxiety—that a misspoken word of prayer would cause his family to lose confidence in him. Although he immediately realized that his fear was irrational, that wasn't enough to wipe it out. So Ethan chose to put the irrational fear right on the Sabbath table—he stated it out loud. His family disproved the fear in a way he would never forget. Amen.

17

PARENTING THE SHY CHILD

Those parents are wise that can fit their nurture according to their nature.

Anne Bradstreet, 1612–1672

It is not easy being a parent these days. We worry about so many catastrophes that might befall our children: accidents, abduction, abuse, and addiction, to name a few. Excessive shyness may seem trivial in comparison, a bit like the smoking habit of a soldier on the front line. But social anxiety is often not benign. Research studies have found that social fears can interfere with the development of social skills and friendships, leading to low self-esteem. Anxious children are less happy and less well liked by their peers, and dating fears can affect a teenager's ability to establish long-term relationships later in life. One study, which followed a group of children into adulthood, showed that extreme shyness led to problems in finding and keeping a good job as well as delays in finding and keeping a marriage partner.

While parents cannot protect their children from every potential catastrophe, parents *can* help with shyness. As their children's first and most important social partners, parents are in a unique position to teach ways to cope with shyness and sometimes to overcome it. Often, by making relatively minor adjustments in their child-rearing style, parents can promote the development of self-esteem and the skills kids will need to thrive in a relentlessly social world.

185

COMMON AND UNCOMMON
SOCIAL FEARS

Some social fears are a normal part of growing up. Fear of unfamiliar people is a stage of development that occurs in most children between six and fifteen months of age. While these fears should not be confused with social anxiety problems, for some children fears persist beyond the normal "stranger anxiety" period and become problematic.

Many of these children seem to have been born shy, to have inherited a shy disposition or temperament. Estimates of what proportion of children are shy vary depending on what cutoff point is used, but a rate of about 15 percent is commonly cited. In chapter 9 we discussed evidence that a shy or inhibited temperament may reflect an inherited tendency of the nervous system to be activated easily by unfamiliar situations or people. Even when shyness has a strong hereditary or physiological component, however, it can still be influenced by parenting approaches.

Husband and wife psychiatrists Stella Chess and Alexander Thomas, in landmark studies that followed thousands of infants into adulthood, described some infants with a "difficult" temperament pattern that included reacting negatively to unfamiliar things. In addition to crying or being bashful in social situations, the "slow-to-warm-up" baby may have difficulty with unfamiliarity in general—for example, rejecting new foods. Later, as a five- or six-year-old, the same child may shy away from other children on the playground, particularly if parents are not actively encouraging group play. By the time this child is ten, his or her lack of experience in approaching other children may have further increased social anxiety.

HOW PARENTS INFLUENCE SHYNESS

The born-shy child poses a challenge to parents. One natural reaction of parents is to protect such a child. Seeing how distressed her child becomes when dealing with aggressive playmates, a mother might try to confront the playmate herself, or might limit visits to the playground in order to "protect" her child. Another common reaction, especially as the child becomes older, might be to criticize the child's shyness and insist that he or she enter social activities. While it is understandable for parents to react in these ways, the slow-to-warm-up baby will do better with a combination of emotional support and exposure to social activity. Later in this chapter we will describe some specific ways for parents to help their shy children.

It is quite common for a shy child to have at least one parent who was also shy as a child or who is still socially anxious. Many such parents worry that their children will learn social fears from them, and there is some basis to this worry. Children are extremely sensitive to their parents' reactions to people, and they learn to use the same methods to deal with their own fears. A parent who fears meeting other parents when she is taking her child to the toddler swim class at the local Y transmits that unease to her child. The child then enters swim class with an elevated sense of danger about this novel social situation. Again, parent and child reinforce each other's nervousness: Child looks fearful, parent overreacts to the child's fear with more worry, and on and on it goes, shaping new social fears.

On the other hand, the life experiences of formerly shy parents may give them a special ability both to empathize with what their child is going through and to recognize the importance of helping their child confront his or her fears. Shy parents often understand firsthand the need to avoid the overprotective behaviors that lead to overdependence. A mother who took her child to summer camp for the first time confessed, "It was very difficult to leave her there. . . . I kept thinking about how nervous I would have been at her age, feeling as if nobody would want to talk with me or be my friend. But I also remembered that I didn't get over my fears until my mother stopped trying to protect me from the world. Facing my fears without her at my side was painful, but I made it. I told my daughter that when I was her age, sometimes it was scary for me to meet new people, but I knew a trick she could use. If she was friendly and showed some interest in people, the ones who really mattered would like her, and she would make some new friends."

Parents who have had their own problems with social fears may find themselves reliving some painful memories as they observe their children struggling with shyness. In such instances, it is important for parents to keep some perspective. Identifying too closely with a child's discomfort may lead a parent to overprotect, but this simply reinforces the child's mistaken belief that social situations are very dangerous, and it denies the child crucial opportunities to learn social skills.

Older children and adolescents who are struggling with social anxiety may recognize the fearful style of a parent as unhelpful and seek out socially bolder individuals as role models. Adolescent boys, in particular, will work hard to avoid being labeled a "mama's boy." Girls, on the other hand, experience less need to avoid being seen as dependent, and they are less likely to go to extremes in declaring their independence. Shy children should be encouraged in their efforts at independence. Sometimes, the best way to help may be to offer less help.

Some parents who are not shy themselves may inadvertently bring out social anxiety in their children through efforts to teach good social behavior. These parents try to teach social skills by admonishing children to avoid behavior that will result in the disapproval of others: "Don't play with your food when we get to Aunt Tasha's house or she'll think you're a baby," "Don't play with the girls or they'll say you're a sissy," and so on.

Children who are bombarded with these types of "shame" tactics may learn to "behave," but they also learn that social encounters are as dangerous as a minefield. Fear of being shamed or embarrassed becomes the major motivation for their behavior, rather than the wish to enjoy contact with others. Another tactic that leads to poor results is the use of strong punishment for a child who avoids a social situation. Studies show that boys who are heavily punished in general by their parents have more problems making and keeping friends.

A different kind of parent-child miscommunication is more subtle, but can be equally troublesome. When five-year-old Tommy cried in the presence of a large group of unfamiliar relatives, his mother, instead of acknowledging his fear, told him: "You're *not* afraid. The Smith family always loves to be around people." Tommy got the confusing message that either he was experiencing something other than fear or he must not be a member of the Smith family. And because Tommy surely wanted to remain a member of the Smith family, he learned to deny his fears and lose touch with his feelings—including the feeling of anger at his mother for rejecting the part of him that was fearful.

Here the parent, in a well-meaning but mistaken effort to help, attempted to do Tommy's emotional homework for him. Learning to recognize and label feelings is a child's first step in dealing with them, a normal part of the process of developing mastery and self-confidence. If Tommy learns that his shy feelings are unacceptable to his family, this lesson will undermine his developing self-esteem, which may already be on the low side.

Recognizing a child's feelings can have the opposite effect. What if his mother had instead said, "Are you feeling scared around all these people? It can be scary at first when you meet a lot of new people, but it helps to find a friend to play with. Let's go meet your cousin Phil, who can be terrific fun.'' First, Tommy would learn that even his disturbing feelings are acceptable to his parents and not a cause for rejection or alarm. He also would learn a label for them, ''being scared,'' which will help him process and manage these emotions. Finally, his mother would have introduced a constructive approach to coping with the feeling that Tommy can eventually learn to put into effect on his own.

RECOGNIZING PROBLEM SHYNESS

But how is a parent to know when the normal socialization process has gone astray? What behaviors in children are signs that mild shyness or a tendency to be bashful has gone too far, moving into the realm of trouble? For example, we know that clinging to Mom at age two or three is normal but that the same behavior at age five, six, or seven is not. Children who are eleven, twelve, or thirteen naturally may be embarrassed by changes in the appearance of their bodies, but if as a result they refuse to change clothes for gym class they are having a significant problem.

While the border between ''normal'' and excessive social anxiety is often unclear, as a rule of thumb normal fears tend to be transient and only mildly distressing to children. The longer a fear persists without improvement, the greater the cause for concern. Fears that interfere with a child's functioning in school or in social activities also signal a problem. Many parents, hoping for the best, tend to assume that their children will outgrow a social anxiety problem. About half of shy and timid toddlers will overcome their fears to a significant degree by age eight, so that they show normal sociability and emotional spontaneity, but half will continue with significant shyness.

Because of the long-term risks attached to serious shyness, it makes sense to err on the side of making an extra effort to help children cope with even mild fears. The following signs are some indicators that further attention is needed and a change in parenting tactics may be helpful.

Common Signs of Excessive Shyness

Sign	Typical Grade
1. Child is easily and persistently frightened by strangers	Preschool (ages 3–5)
2. Child constantly clings to parent in public situations, like grocery store or at other person's home	Preschool to third grade
3. Child refuses to speak, especially in school	Especially preschool to fourth grade
4. Child frequently complains of being sick in order to stay home from school	Especially K–fourth grade
5. Child refuses to go to school	K–eighth grade
6. Child has few or no friends	All grades
7. Child skips gym class or forgets gym clothes to avoid changing in front of others	Sixth–eighth grade
8. Child spends a great deal of time alone in room	Especially sixth–twelfth grade
9. Child does not date and does not attend social group activities	High school
10. Child spends an excessive amount of time engaged in solo ''electronic'' activities like Nintendo, TV, computer games	Fifth–twelfth grade
11. Child becomes extremely anxious when taking tests	All grades
12. Child is afraid to speak up in class	All grades

No one sign indicates that your child is in trouble, of course, and shyness is not the only explanation for the above signs. For example, a child's refusal to go to school may be due to being picked on by the neighborhood bully or to problems with a teacher, rather than a social phobia.

When a parent detects a possible warning sign, the first step is to try to confirm whether the nature of the problem is social anxiety or something else. Regarding the younger child, this may mean paying more attention to his or her behavior with peers. It may also be helpful to find out if a teacher or the parent of a playmate has noticed any problems, such as a tendency to steer away from group activities or games.

Asking your child about his feelings or reasons for any of these

Children Who Won't Talk

A small number of children show the extreme avoidant behavior of never speaking up in certain situations outside the home—for example, by remaining silent at school. This condition, recently termed "selective mutism," is more common in girls, usually begins in early childhood, and may be brief or persistent until the teenage years. Selective mutism typically gets recognized as a problem when the child starts school, and it alarms teachers and parents.

Selective mutism has been very difficult to study and explain because these children usually refuse to speak to therapists as well. It was once believed that many of these children must have suffered extreme trauma or family problems. Recent studies, however, based on interviews with parents and teachers (and yes-or-no answers from children willing to respond with nods and shakes of the head) suggest a strong connection to social anxiety. These children, when they do speak, sometimes report that their voices sound funny and that they don't want others to hear their voices.

Information about which treatments are most effective is limited. A few studies have shown positive results with cognitive-behavioral therapy, including gradual exposure to difficult speaking situations combined with praise and rewards for increasing amounts of talking. Some success with Prozac and other medications has also been reported. The appendix lists additional sources of information on selective mutism.

behaviors is certainly worth a try, but for a variety of reasons it may be a dead end. Most six-year-olds cannot clearly define "embarrassment," although by age eight they have usually developed the ability to put this emotion into words. Teenagers have the vocabulary to describe their social anxiety, but they may be too insecure to admit these feelings to their parents. Whether the anxiety gets discussed or not, an essential component of any parenting approach is empathy—trying to put yourself in the child's shoes. After observing and collecting information, a parent may try some new approaches on for size.

HOW TO HELP

So what is a parent to do about a shy child? As one colleague put it, "Parents need to take a firm stand . . . right in the middle." It is important to "walk the line" between extreme actions, such as forcing a child to play with others (as if a child could be forced to play!), and sheltering a child from social fears by removing the child from every uncomfortable encounter. The challenge for parents is to discover a means to help their children gradually increase social activity and ability without forcing them in a way that leads to tremendous discomfort and greater fear.

The concepts involved in helping children cope with shyness are basically the same as those that can help adults. See chapter 15 for a constructive step-by-step approach to accomplishing specific goals. Parents can use the same general approach to plan ways of coaching their children in coping with shyness. Of course, using the method with children requires some special considerations, as we will discuss below.

For younger children (under age twelve), parents need to focus on changing social behaviors rather than on trying to change fearful thinking, because these children are still developing the capacity to think abstractly about their fears. Improvement in the child's fearful thinking will follow. Because the young child cannot see the long-term benefits of the short-term anxiety that comes with confronting feared situations, parents need to provide the motivation. One way parents can encourage younger children is to reward modest achievements in their social program. For example, a child could receive a sticker on a "star chart" for accomplishing weekly goals, with a certain number of stickers earning small prizes or special privileges. Social exercises can be turned into more palatable games.

A STEP-BY-STEP APPROACH

Parents should start by setting reasonable goals. The seven-year-old girl who is fearful about speaking up in front of her class for show-and-tell should not be expected to perform so well as to win the lead role in *Annie*. Nor should she be allowed to refuse to go to school on show-and-tell days. A parent's assistance package for show-and-tell fears might consist of the following steps:

1. Set a goal. ("I think you'll feel good about your show-and-tell if you can *tell your class three fun things about your project*.")

2. Help your child to be prepared. (Rehearse by having your child give the presentation with you playing the audience.)

3. Make supportive, positive comments about the presentation and your confidence in your child's abilities. ("You really do have something great to say!" "I know you can do it ... just like you did last week when you told a story in class.")

4. Avoid making too big a deal about the presentation.

5. After the presentation is done, briefly review how it went. ("Did you talk about your project?")

6. Praise any behavior that comes close to the goal. ("You were able to get up there and talk to your whole class.")

Before setting a goal, first recognize what your child is already able to do, such as being able to tell her friends about her project. In selecting goals, choose specific behaviors that your child is likely to be able to accomplish (here, saying just a few things about her project). The point is to insure success in order to build confidence, not to try to make great leaps in social abilities. Also, when setting goals, avoid trying to control uncontrollable emotions such as nervousness. For example, don't set a goal such as "I will do my show-and-tell without getting nervous" or "I will feel good about my talk." Focus on what the child needs to do rather than on how she should feel. Good feelings will follow success.

Being prepared is also important. Children will want to avoid practicing behaviors that make them anxious. The parent must shoulder responsibility for making a rehearsal happen. ("Bring your spelling words here so we can practice for your spelling bee" or "Go and get your show-and-tell project so we can practice your speech.") Parent and child can take turns being the presenter or the audience. This allows the parent to "model" certain behaviors that may be missing from the child's repertoire (like speaking clearly or making eye contact with audience members). The parent should provide feedback that emphasizes what the child did well. (''You did the first part real well. Now let's try the second part again'' or ''Your introduction was awesome. Let's think of a few more things you can say about your project.'')

Once you have finished setting performance goals, rehearsing the event, and providing positive feedback about the child's performance during rehearsal, it's a good idea to avoid hyping the importance of the upcoming event. By having focused on adequate preparation, but not making a big deal about the upcoming performance, the parent transmits the message that what is important has already transpired: ''You are ready for this, and you can 'put the event away in a box' for now.'' Obsessing about what might go wrong is unproductive and will only fuel fear and anxiety. Instead, review the coping plan briefly or move on to other activities.

In a similar fashion, the parent should try to remain laid-back in processing the event once it is over. An easygoing ''How did it go today?'' might be followed by a brief reminder of the original goal. Children (and adults) will usually forget about the original goal and instead comment on how they were feeling during the event. ''I was nervous'' should be followed by the response ''That's natural, but what about your goal? You remember, your goal to tell the class those three things.'' The child's response—''Yeah, I guess I made my goal''—should be followed by positive remarks from the parent: ''That's great. I knew it was going to be tough, but I also knew that you could accomplish it.''

USING REWARDS EFFECTIVELY

In real life, many opportunities to make social gains will crop up quickly, leaving you little time to plan or to walk through the preliminary steps mentioned above. Regardless of the situation, the key to success is to focus on positive aspects of your child's performance. As any good schoolteacher knows, ''Catch me when I'm good'' is the guiding principle for shaping desired behaviors in children. Reward your child's attempts to approach other children in the playground, to invite other children to your house, or to sign up for after-school activities. Use positive talk (''That's terrific how you invited Sheila to your party'') or tangible rewards, such as a milk-and-cookies treat with Mom or Dad.

At first, when trying to shape a new behavior such as approaching other children at the playground, it is a good idea to praise or reward your child *each time* she or he returns from having made an attempt to join others. During this period of "continuous reinforcement," praise or rewards should be delivered immediately and with sincerity. The closer the proximity of the praise to the behavior, the more powerful its effect. Once approaching other children becomes a regular part of your child's social repertoire, shift to a more intermittent delivery of positive attention. Deliver your verbal praise or tangible goody once in a while, rather than each time you observe the desired behavior. Such intermittent reward is particularly powerful and helps to "seal in" new social behaviors.

Once you see that your child is approaching other children with regularity and is experiencing the natural reinforcement of enjoying play, you may decide to move on to another important behavior. You might now select a verbal behavior goal, such as talking nicely to other children. Studies in child psychology have illuminated differences between the successful and unsuccessful child on the playground. The successful child asks questions ("Can I play?" or "What game are you playing?"), while the unsuccessful child makes statements ("I know how to play" or "I'm going to play, too"). Parents can help by demonstrating effective questions for breaking the ice and by reinforcing the kind of talk that will lead to positive experiences.

The important thing to keep in mind when deciding which behaviors to "shape up" is to "start small." Take your cue from what your child can already do from time to time and build on his or her strengths. So, if your child never speaks to adults, but does occasionally look up at them, you may choose to reward appropriately longer eye contact with adults ... or to simply reward hanging out in close proximity to adults. Shaping a new behavior is much like shaping a clay figure ... you start with something that looks nothing like the end product. But gradually you "shape" it so that it begins to look like what you had desired.

Of course, the behaviors you select for shaping should be appropriate for your child and for your child's age. One mother we know, in an unintentionally misguided twist on *My Fair Lady,* felt compelled to tutor her eight-year-old son in the chivalrous arts of holding doors open for girls in his class and walking between a girl and the street. Her son recognized the irrelevance of these behaviors and simply refused to cooperate.

Examples of how some parents approached their own children's unique situations and made these techniques their own follow.

ARRANGING BUT NOT PUSHING

A formerly shy parent of an extremely shy five-year-old recently told us, "I never push Emily to talk or play . . . because I hated when my mother did that to me." What she does do is constantly *arrange* for the possibility of social exposure opportunities for her daughter. She brings Emily along on weekend sales calls so that she can get used to meeting other adults. She takes Emily to the playground (but doesn't force her to play with other children). In the summer, she takes her frequently to the town beach or to the public library for group storytelling events. In sum, she simultaneously encourages social activity, naturally cuts down on escape routes (it's hard not to interact with other children at these places), and respects her daughter's wishes to cling to her sometimes or to play by herself.

This mother usually discovers that Emily holds back at first but eventually becomes interested in what others are up to. In her own time, the child begins to "play around the edge" of others, and sometimes becomes directly "taken in" by other children's play activities. In her mother's words, "Emily has a different social rhythm . . . she needs more time to warm up to others." Adopting this approach means accepting the fact that there will be times when your child will not warm up and will choose instead to avoid contact with others—and that's okay!

One way to know whether to push or to arrange opportunities is by looking at your own record of results. Does a gentle push with a word of encouragement work, or does it lead to resistance or clinging? There is a tendency for parents to push *even harder* when gentle pushing has failed. This approach usually leads to misery for both parent and child: the child hunkers down and keeps resisting; the parent cajoles, pleads, and eventually yells. The lesson from this "cycle of pain" is clear: Stop pushing and shift to less heavy-handed arranging.

Some parents have told us that pushing has been effective in helping their children get started. From the time Jesse was a young child, his parents would push him to join all sorts of social activities, from after-school sports to group music lessons and the school marching band. He would briefly whine and try to make excuses for not going, but once he got into it, he had a great time . . . so his parents continued to push him. Now a medical student, Jesse says he still agonizes over making telephone calls or visiting a professor's office: "It's just like when I was a kid . . . but once I jump into the situation, everything goes just fine.... The only difference between now and then is that as an adult I have to push myself.''

ARRANGING AND REINFORCING: "MELISSA GOES TO THE LIBRARY"

Marilyn's five-year-old daughter was so shy that Marilyn would feel guilty whenever she took her out in public. Melissa looked pained whenever she unexpectedly had to greet adults or children. One day, a neighbor who had a daughter the same age encouraged Marilyn to bring Melissa to the storytelling program at the local public library. While Marilyn knew that Melissa would likely become anxious about joining a large group of strangers, she knew that it was important to get Melissa out of the house and into friendly, low-key situations where she could meet other people.

When Marilyn informed her daughter of a plan to visit the library one Saturday morning, she made a point of "hyping" the event, exclaiming that there was going to be an "awesome story" and that they could go out for ice cream afterward with the neighbor and her daughter. When Melissa began to complain mildly about having to go, Marilyn told her that she didn't have to play with anyone, that her goal was simply to sit through at least one story. In the hour leading up to their departure for the library, Melissa would occasionally whine about going: "Do we *have* to go?" or "I'm gonna miss *Muppet Babies* on TV." Her mother said she would respond to talk but not to whining. Marilyn was careful to *ignore* whining and to attend instead to any talk that was in a more appropriate tone.

During story time at the library, Melissa would move between clinging to her mother and sitting up front with other children listening to the story. Marilyn told her daughter once that she would hear the story better and have more fun if she sat up front. After that, Marilyn ignored her clinging but made no effort to push her away or otherwise force her to sit with other children. The "communication" of Mom's behavior was clear: "You are allowed to hide behind me if you wish, but I am not going to shower you with affection if you've come to cling." Melissa soon found that the social goodies lay not with Mom but up front with the other children.

Overall, Marilyn found this tactic to be useful. She took advantage of free or low-cost children's events (such as birthday parties and activities at the local children's museum or at the public library), but she never pushed her child to interact with others. Simultaneously, she rewarded (by her praise and attention) the types of talk and play that she wanted to see more of in Melissa, and she tended to ignore the ones that she wanted to see less often.

The technique of ignoring unwanted behaviors is not a form of punishment and should not be done angrily. Ignoring is instead a type of "delay tactic" that signals to the child that praise and reward are not available under the current circumstances, but that praise and reward will be available as soon as better behaviors occur. While the parent can state this policy up front, following through with action is most important. If a child becomes frustrated or even throws tantrums in response to this approach, it is then especially important to persist until the child switches to a more acceptable behavior. Any premature shift to providing attention will have the unwanted effect of strengthening undesirable behaviors such as whining and clinging.

A CAVEAT ON NAGGING

Shy kids of all ages, like children who misbehave, are constantly prompted, or told what to do, by their parents: "Go play with Andrea," "You need to get out of your room," "You need to stop hanging around the house." Parents verbally direct these children literally hundreds of times each day—*even though it doesn't work!* Of course, it's understandable for parents to feel frustrated when they see that their shy children are missing out on desirable social activities. Unfortunately, frustration doesn't often lead to effective problem solving. Instead, we often lean harder on what is already not working with the idea that if we push just a little harder . . . Well, imagine if someone told you what to do a few hundred times each day. After a while, these instructions would lose their effectiveness. For the child, having Mom and Dad repeat themselves over and over again beats having to do whatever they might be requesting.

The solution is simple: stop nagging. We recommend that you adopt "the rule of two," which simply states that a parent should never repeat an instruction more than once. This follows the principle that instructions are only useful if people follow them. If your child complies with your prompt, seize the opportunity to reward that response by heaping on the praise. If your child does not comply, try once more, but change your language, this time inserting the word *need* in your request: "I *need* you to go outside and greet your cousins," or "You *need* to say hello to your Uncle Herb." If you are consistent, the word *need* will now become a cue to the child that this is the final request. Failure to comply this time should reliably lead to some small negative consequence, such as the loss of a privilege, a fifteen-minute earlier bedtime, or an allowance reduction. This method is tough but effective.

FEARS OF THE MIDDLE SCHOOL YEARS AND BEYOND

A child's social pressures begin to spiral upward sometime around the sixth grade. Boys and girls become more aware of sexuality and pressures to be "cool" or "in" or "popular" begin to mount. At this age, children begin to feel less understood by their parents, and they are often correct. Parents will make flip remarks or joke that their children have a girlfriend or boyfriend. In many cases, they ignore the social changes their children are going through altogether. But make no mistake about it, these are painful times for many kids, and especially for shy ones.

These are also tough times for parents. They see their children becoming more independent and disconnected, and attempts to keep lines of communication open may be rebuffed. Combine this break between parent and child with adolescent social anxiety, and both parties are left with an extremely challenging situation. At this age socially anxious children may begin to feel hopeless. They see themselves as social failures *and* feel uncomfortable talking about their feelings with their parents. This mixture of insecurity, alienation, and social humiliation can be a recipe for depression and even thoughts of suicide. It is important for parents to persist in maintaining communication even in the absence of encouragement from these children.

Megan was always seen as a happy and content child until she reached sixth grade. Natalie, her closest friend since the first grade, began to hang out with a different group of kids and made no attempt to invite Megan to join in. Megan tried repeatedly to reconnect with Natalie by calling her or by inviting her over after school. Natalie, going along with her new group's thinking that Megan was no longer "cool," however, ignored Megan's attempts to stay friends.

Megan felt humiliated by the rejection of Natalie and the other kids, and she began isolating herself at home. By the seventh grade, Megan began to experience extreme anxiety whenever she came into contact with children her own age. She began to complain frequently of physical problems, often pleading with her parents to allow her to stay home from school. Although her parents made endless attempts to talk with Megan about her problems, she limited her responses to talking about how she felt physically: "I can't go to school because my throat is killing me!" Only after Megan established a connection with a therapist was she able to tie her physical pains to her fears of being rejected by her peers at school.

The ability to use words and talking therapy grows with age. Very young children may not understand the words that describe their problem or explain possible solutions. They need their parents to recognize their experience and to help put it into words. If a parent has been able to acknowledge and accept the child's fears in the past, the growing child will find it easier to recognize new fears when they occur and will feel less shame over them. Fears that are "out on the table" become much easier to address.

Awareness of fears is very much a part of the experience of social anxiety in teenagers. This is an age at which children's behavior is falling less and less under the influence of parental "arranging." Fortunately, the adolescent's growing ability to reflect on his anxious thinking also brings the capacity to learn new and more sophisticated skills for coping with social skills.

Parents can help adolescents use the same kind of cognitive-behavioral self-help approach that we described in chapter 15. As in adults, a plan for behavior change in teenagers can be supported and reinforced by self-talk. Parents can help teach the concept that *a fearful thought is not a fact*. Instead, a fear is an idea or theory that can be analyzed and questioned. It can be challenged head-on in a supportive way: "What would actually happen if you messed up your speech, and how bad would it really be? What are the real odds that your fear that everyone will walk out would come true? Would you walk out on a speaker just because he or she seemed anxious? Would some people be impressed that you were up there at all?"

Through this process your child can learn to recognize that the fearful thought is an exaggeration, and that by looking at the situation more realistically, it becomes easier to handle. What started as a frightening "I'll blow the talk and everyone will think I'm a jerk" becomes a reassuring "I'll get my ideas across, and people I care about will respect me for trying." If your teenager is willing to discuss, for example, fears about dating, briefly pursuing fearful thoughts can be helpful:

TEENAGER: Next week is the prom? . . . I don't think I'm gonna go.
  PARENT: (makes light inquiry) Oh?
     TEEN: I was thinking of asking Stephanie . . . but I don't think she would go with me.

PARENT: Are you absolutely sure that she wouldn't?

TEEN: Well, no ... I suppose she might say yes ... but she might say no.

PARENT: So what if she says no? Could you handle that?

TEEN: I'd probably be the laughingstock of the whole school.

PARENT: *Everyone* would laugh at you? You mean everybody else gets a date to the prom?

TEEN: Not everyone, I suppose.... Kevin and Kyle aren't going—maybe we can hold an alternative prom for dorks!

PARENT: (jokingly) I could provide the calculators and pencil holders!

Instead of countering the teen's fears by saying they were not true, this parent *asked questions* that helped the teen come to rational conclusions *on his own*. In this situation, the parent could have taken a variety of avenues in pursuing fears and presenting alternative ideas ("How would you feel if you didn't ask Stephanie out and it turned out she had been interested in going?" or "If Stephanie turns down your offer, are there any other girls you might ask?"). Often, if you pursue an idea for which your teen is entertaining a catastrophic ending, he or she will at least realize that the consequences are not so severe and that even worst-case scenarios, such as being rejected for a prom date, are manageable.

META TALK: TALKING ABOUT TALKING

While it's important for parents to talk to their kids about problems they notice, a more sensitive child may resist parents' attempts at pursuing fearful ideas about social encounters. While your initial impulse as a parent may be to walk away and avoid being intrusive, another tactic is to approach the topic indirectly by "talking about having that conversation." The parent might ask, "What would it be like if we were to talk about the prom?" as opposed to asking directly about the prom. Talking with your child this way may seem odd, especially if you have never tried it, but if the alternative is silence, you have little to lose. The teen might respond by saying that it might be embarrassing to talk about it, and in a short time might begin to talk more directly. The parent moves carefully from the outside in.

Meta-conversations allow parents to enter a dialogue with a child by acknowledging that a topic is difficult to discuss. Asking a teen "What would it be like to talk with your old man about sex?" is different from saying "I need to ask you questions about your current sexual activities." Similarly, "What would it be like for you to join the after-school theater group?" differs from the more threatening "You must join this group if you are ever to make any friends" and gradually sets the stage for talking about the real thing.

One parent suspected that his son had become depressed and withdrawn over lacking a date for the homecoming game. He feared he might humiliate his son if he asked him about it directly. At the same time, he sensed that his son needed someone to talk to about his disappointment. Their meta-conversation went something like this:

FATHER: (casually sits next to his seventeen-year-old son on living room couch) Howzit going, Danny?
TEEN: (doesn't look up)   Huh?
FATHER: You look a bit down. . . . I was wondering how it's going.
TEEN: I'm okay.
FATHER: Oh, good . . . I was a little worried. Would it be all right if I asked you what might be bugging you a little bit? Or would that be too weird to talk about with your dad?
TEEN: (half smiling) It would probably be a little weird.
FATHER: Any weirder than when we had that talk about what was bothering you a few months ago?
TEEN: No, that was no big deal.

Up until this point, the focus of this father-and-son conversation is on having a conversation about out-of-the-ordinary topics. The father is making a slow but effective entry into talking about his son's problem even though neither has mentioned it directly. To the father's surprise, his son is the first one to bring up the topic:

TEEN: This isn't that big a deal either, Dad. . . . I was just hoping that me and Claire would go to the homecoming game together.
FATHER: Oh . . . what happened?
TEEN: Nothing . . . I'm pretty sure that she's gonna go with someone else.
FATHER: Oh, that's too bad. . . . Are you sure?

By simultaneously respecting his son's right to privacy and asking if it is all right to broach a difficult topic, the father has succeeded in engaging his son in a conversation about the problem. While setting the stage for a conversation about his son's disappointment may not solve his fear of asking someone to the game, it at least opens up the possibility of help by spurring on productive problem solving. By asking the question ''Are you sure [that Claire won't go with you to the game]?'' the father at least introduces the concept of questioning the accuracy of anxious thoughts. Dad was surprised again by his son's response:

> TEEN: (looks up) I'm not absolutely sure . . . but she's, like, incredibly popular.
>
> FATHER: What would it be like for you to ask her to the game?
>
> TEEN: I would get real nervous just asking her . . . she'd think I was a jerk.
>
> FATHER: Are we both talking about the Claire who lives next door? You guys have been friends since we moved to Fergus Falls. Do you really think she would think you were a jerk for asking her to the game?
>
> TEEN: Well, she might not think I'm a jerk, but it would be embarrassing . . .
>
> FATHER: If Claire says no, is there anybody else you think you might ask?
>
> TEEN: Yeah, Amy and Melinda told me they want to go . . .
>
> FATHER: (kiddingly) Gee, in the old days you would take me to the games. . . . Remember the year Fergus made it to the Otter County championship? . . .

By the end of the conversation, the teenager is equipped with the useful perspective that it wouldn't be the end of the world if Claire said no. He also feels emotionally supported by his father, saying in essence, ''I'm glad that you'll be here if I get knocked off the ladder.'' The father gains something also. He sees that taking a little bit of time and utilizing a meta-talk strategy can help him maintain an all-important communication link to his teenage son. On the negative side, Dad still needs to curb his tendency to cut serious conversations short by changing the topic, which probably result from his own social anxiety.

Finally, there are times when despite a parent's best intentions, a child is unwilling to talk about social fears and problems. Rather than forcing a conversation, try again at a later time. This is where a parent must be creative in order to give the child ''permission'' to talk about the issue.

USING ALCOHOL TO "SELF-MEDICATE"

Most American teens discover alcohol before age sixteen. Some try it and are not captivated by its effects. Others, unfortunately, immediately discover that it has temporary anxiety-relieving effects for them. The scenario is all too common: The teen with social fears is offered beer or wine at a party and finds that social anxiety dissipates. The party may become more than just "manageable." The tipsy teen may even be thrilled to experience this window of freedom from anxiety. Alcohol (and other drug use) becomes a powerful reinforcer, increasing the likelihood that the teen will seek it out again and again, even after the social relief no longer occurs. Ultimately, the solution will not lie in parents' simply forbidding the teen from going out or attending parties, but instead will require helping the teen learn to manage social situations in ways other than using alcohol.

WHEN TO SEEK PROFESSIONAL HELP

A persistent drug or alcohol problem in a child is one obvious sign that professional therapy is needed. The same holds true for other serious complications of social anxiety, such as depression or school avoidance. But a parent shouldn't wait for a crisis to seek help or at least to get an evaluation of the need for help by a professional. If a child seems consistently distressed or is stuck with persistent social anxiety problems that don't respond to the simple measures we have outlined, a consultation can head off future complications or can even ultimately be life-saving.

After this review of all that can go wrong in the development of self-esteem, social skills, and relationships, it may seem miraculous that any parent can guide a child through this gauntlet. Fortunately, it all works out more often than not. Most parents know their children better than any book can say, and children are remarkably resilient in meeting the inevitable social challenges of life. For most kids, social anxiety problems are temporary, and when they do persist, there is more than one right way to cope with them.

VI

TREATMENT FOR SOCIAL PHOBIA

18

PSYCHOLOGICAL THERAPIES

Why dost thou not speak? queried one.
'Tis that people stare so, I replied.
It maketh my heart to flutter,
my breath to pant, and
my tongue to stutter.
'Twould be death to continue, I cried.

Nay, they said, thou be a fool.
Assuredly thou dramatize thy plight
Speak, and thou wilt find favour
In other's sight.
They lied ... I died!

Lucinda Scott-Smith, 1994

Most people with social anxiety problems, like the poet above, are familiar with the experience of receiving well-intended but unhelpful advice from friends and family. In the past, many psychotherapy approaches used by professionals were also of limited or unknown benefit to people with social phobia. More recently, however, therapy approaches specifically designed for social phobia have proved effective in research studies and tremendously helpful to individual sufferers. In this chapter, we will discuss some of the psychological therapies in common use for social phobia, focusing on those with the most evidence of being effective, and we will examine some practical issues involved in finding a therapist.

COGNITIVE-BEHAVIORAL THERAPIES

The best established psychological therapies for social phobia have grown out of the science of cognitive-behavioral psychology. In this form of treatment, the therapist takes an active stance, asking specific questions to determine which situations are problematic and what the person actually thinks and does in these situations. The therapist serves as both a teacher and a coach, helping to identify problem behaviors and thinking patterns and to develop more effective coping strategies. Opportunities to practice these new strategies are planned, and the therapist provides feedback about how the person's efforts are going. Unlike traditional psychotherapy, cognitive-behavioral therapy does not attempt to search for the original causes of the problem, because understanding the cause is usually not essential for change, and it would rob time from efforts to build new behaviors.

Cognitive-behavioral approaches that were first developed to treat depression have recently been adapted specifically for problems with social anxiety. Among the psychologists who have taken the lead in developing cognitive-behavioral therapies for social phobia are Richard Heimberg, who developed group therapy programs, and Samuel Turner and Deborah Beidel, who focused on combined individual and group behavior therapy and social skills training.

In the late 1980s, Heimberg showed that a therapy that taught groups of patients how to develop more realistic views of their social abilities and used role playing to allow for practice of new coping skills was helpful in reducing social anxiety. A participant in Heimberg's cognitive-behavioral group therapy can expect to practice directly confronting social fears (starting with the mildest ones), typically in weekly two-hour sessions over a period of twelve weeks. Each group member selects a social or public situation that is anxiety producing, such as speaking up at a party or making a sales pitch at a business meeting. With the help of one of the therapists (ideally, there are two), each member writes a list of his or her fearful thoughts ("Nobody will want to talk to me at the party"). The accuracy of these thoughts is challenged on a rational basis, and alternative coping phrases are developed ("I have several interesting things to tell people").

Therapists then help arrange a series of role plays designed to simulate the feared situation of each group member in turn. Other group members take various roles in these exercises, such as playing audience members for a speech, potential customers during a sales pitch, or partygoers for an attempt to initiate conversation. The group member enters the simulation with a preplanned goal in mind ("I will introduce myself and bring up at least one topic of conversation to others at the 'party' "). The therapist signals that the role play is to begin, and the main actor utters his or her coping phrases and begins a five-minute simulation of the feared situation. Afterward, the therapist leads a discussion in which group members discuss the outcome of the role play and give the main actor feedback on the performance. Each group member leaves the session with homework tasks involving exposure to real-life situations that are to be attempted outside of the office. As the group members master their least difficult situations, they move on to more challenging ones.

Several research studies have clearly established the effectiveness of this type of cognitive-behavioral group therapy (or CBGT) by comparing it with nonspecific treatments. Researchers use nonspecific treatments to control for the possibility that subjects might improve due to chance, due to the attention or enthusiasm of the therapists, or through some other mechanism beside the specific effects of CBGT. This series of studies has shown that twelve weeks of CBGT is more effective than putting subjects on a waiting list (which controls for chance improvement), more effective than a group treatment consisting of emotional support and education about anxiety (but no cognitive-behavioral techniques), and more effective than a "sugar pill" placebo (which subjects believed could have been an antianxiety medicine). CBGT subjects showed clear improvement in ratings by patients and therapists—and also by independent assessors who were unaware of which treatment each subject had received.

The improvement in symptoms has also been shown to continue at three and six months after treatment has ended, which suggests that people continue to apply the therapy techniques on their own. A follow-up study of nineteen of these participants five years after treatment showed that those who had received CBGT maintained an advantage over those who had received the control therapy. Because the number of persons contacted five years later was quite small, however, the question of long-term effectiveness needs further study.

During the same period in which Heimberg was testing CBGT, Samuel Turner and Deborah Beidel were developing a four-month intensive therapy program they called social effectiveness therapy (SET). The SET program is similar to CBGT in that it involves daily practice of feared social activities. It differs from CBGT in that it lacks the therapy component of directly addressing negative thinking patterns and instead adds a component of teaching social skills, such as how to give a talk or establish a friendship. It also employs an exposure technique called flooding, in which an individual enters (or imagines entering) a highly feared situation and stays in the situation (or imagines staying in the situation) until his anxiety level decreases by at least 50 percent.

In one study, 84 percent of a group of people with social phobia made significant improvement using the SET program. Another study found that twenty sessions of the flooding exposure component alone proved more helpful than a sugar pill placebo, and exposure was also more helpful than a medication treatment (which proved ineffective for social phobia). Some other researchers around the world have reported similar success with their own versions of cognitive-behavioral therapy of social phobia. In summary, the evidence for effectiveness of these therapies for social phobia is convincing, and ongoing research is focusing on fine-tuning these and other versions of cognitive-behavioral treatments by identifying which components are most important.

GROUP VERSUS INDIVIDUAL THERAPY AND OTHER VARIATIONS

Group and individual therapy methods each have certain advantages and disadvantages. One advantage of the group approach is that most group members find it a tremendous relief to learn that other people with social phobia actually exist and even appear normal. Often an immediate bond is formed as members relate to each other's difficulties. Equally important, because the situation of meeting with a group of strangers brings out the fears of social phobic people, the group is a powerful setting in which to work on these exposed fears. Exposures to feared situations—such as giving talks in public or mingling at a party—that can only be imagined in individual therapy can easily be simulated in the group. Individuals benefit from the feedback about their own behavior that they receive from other group members. Finally, group therapies tend to be less expensive than individual therapy.

There are also some drawbacks to the group approach. For many socially anxious people, the prospect of tackling a problem under the scrutiny of a roomful of strangers has all the appeal of a root canal. For this reason, some people prefer to work individually with a therapist, or to begin therapy on an individual basis and then to move on to a group setting once they are more comfortable with the idea. Groups also tend to be more time-consuming, because part of each session focuses on the needs of other group members, and individuals do not get as much direct attention from the therapist as they might in individual therapy. Individual therapy also allows for intermingling into the therapy other personal issues that might be outside the framework of the social phobia group. Finally, individual cognitive-behavioral treatment is far more available than specialized social phobia therapy groups.

Many variations of the cognitive-behavioral therapy, although not as rigorously tested as the specific approaches outlined above, may be equally effective options. Some therapists will use office time to discuss negative thinking styles or general problems in managing social situations and relationships, leaving actual exposure to feared situations to be done on the person's own time, outside of the office. An increasing number of psychiatrists are combining medication treatment with this type of homework-based cognitive-behavioral therapy.

TRADITIONAL PSYCHOTHERAPIES

Some people with social phobia benefit from more traditional therapies. These include insight-oriented or psychoanalytic therapies, which focus on uncovering the unconscious roots of a person's fears, and supportive psychotherapy, in which an empathic and encouraging therapist helps the person sort out interpersonal problems. In each of these approaches, the person develops a working relationship with a supportive, accepting therapist, and the very process of establishing such a relationship may be therapeutic in itself.

In insight-oriented therapies, the therapist may play a less active role, allowing the person to make associations between current problems and feelings, childhood experiences, and aspects of the ongoing relationship between patient and therapist. Unconscious feelings that underlie the anxiety symptoms can be accessed, interpreted, and understood. Discovering an explanation for how social fears developed helps relieve excessive self-blame for failings. These therapies may help restore confidence, thereby indirectly helping people to enter their feared situations and to see them as less threatening.

A risk of traditional therapies, however, is that by emphasizing the search for the roots of the problem, which may take months or years to uncover, they can inadvertently give patients another reason to postpone exposing themselves to their feared situations. In any therapy, such exposure is ultimately necessary for recovery. Some therapists combine traditional insight-oriented or psychoanalytic approaches with cognitive-behavioral therapy. These therapists believe that developing insight into the underlying causes of social problems can aid in the development of more rational thinking and can encourage exposure to feared situations.

The effectiveness of these therapies, unlike the cognitive-behavioral therapies, has not been studied for people with social phobia. Long-term psychotherapies, such as psychoanalytic psychotherapy, are notoriously difficult to assess in a scientifically controlled way. Their effectiveness is supported by relatively weaker evidence of theory and case reports of success.

RELAXATION THERAPIES

Relaxation therapies have also been shown to be helpful for reducing some forms of anxiety. According to Joseph Wolpe, a pioneer in the use of relaxation therapies, the opposite of anxiety is relaxed muscles. Put simply, if your muscles are relaxed, you can't be nervous about anything. One common type of relaxation therapy is called progressive muscle relaxation. Developed in the 1920s by a physician named Jacobson, this method involves systematically tensing and relaxing muscle groups throughout the body, from the toes to the top of the head. Another type of relaxation therapy focuses on exercises to regulate breathing.

Although there is an abundance of research showing that relaxation techniques are useful for reducing overall tension and anxiety, only a few studies have applied it directly to social anxiety. These studies suggest that muscle relaxation is most helpful when the technique is actively used during anxiety-producing social situations, as opposed to when it is practiced only at home or in a therapist's office. Many cognitive-behavioral psychologists use it as one of several tools for fighting anxiety and panic. Other related techniques, such as biofeedback (which involves learning personal control over bodily activities such as heart rate or skin temperature) or meditation (which typically involves concentrating on breathing while repeating certain words or phrases), can also be helpful. Just as with muscle relaxation techniques, biofeedback and meditation alone will rarely be sufficient to manage social anxiety effectively.

ALTERNATIVE THERAPIES

In recent years people have shown an increased interest in alternatives to mainstream therapies for a variety of physical and psychological problems. While the effectiveness of such therapies for social phobia has been little studied, some alternative therapies are commonly used to alleviate social fears.

The Alexander technique is a type of physical therapy that originated in England and is particularly popular among actors and musicians. This approach is based on the premise that anxieties about performing are linked to problems in physical movement and posture. The goal of the therapy is to relieve anxiety by retraining people to position their bodies in natural ways. While one study showed that musicians using the Alexander technique could reduce blood pressure just prior to a concert performance, adequate scientific studies to prove its effectiveness have yet to be done.

Like the Alexander technique, dance movement therapy is based on the idea that there is a connection between movement and emotions. Dance movement therapists examine how a person moves and analyze the type of "flow" of muscle movement. "Tension flow" refers to flow that is bound up like a compressed spring and is said to result in high anxiety and social inhibition. Movement is "free-flowing" when muscles are unrestrained, producing a release of tensions and anxiety, and disinhibition. In dance movement therapy, the person seeking help talks about his or her problems while learning to move in new tension-reducing ways.

In psychodrama, you go onstage with fellow group members surrounding you as supporting cast members and with your therapist sitting in the director's chair, barking out commands and suggestions. The term "role-playing" came from this treatment, which was developed by J. L. Moreno in the 1920s. As with cognitive-behavioral group therapy, psychodrama involves rehearsal and acting out fearful situations, but the therapist analyzes problems very differently, focusing on early childhood experiences.

SELF-HELP GROUPS

The power of self-help groups should not be underestimated. According to a recent review of effective psychotherapies by *Consumer Reports,* the majority of people attending self-help groups for a variety of problems report being highly satisfied. Self-help groups are not intended to take the place of professional evaluation and therapy, but they can provide valuable opportunities to practice social skills and to share emotional support. Any activity that encourages people to get into social situations may supplement professional therapy by providing an opportunity to put into action new coping skills.

Organizations such as the Anxiety Disorders Association of America maintain registries of support groups that are geared toward people with anxiety problems (see the appendix). Groups that focus on coping with social anxiety or on developing social skills may be particularly useful. Toastmasters, an international organization that sponsors public speaking practice groups, can be helpful as a supplement to therapy for public speaking anxiety, and classes on public speaking, acting, or social skills can similarly be useful. The opportunities to practice social skills are endless, ranging from hiking clubs to church activities to political organizations.

A sympathetic or supportive friend, or an informal self-help group in the church basement, has helped a good many people shed some anxiety. Twin brothers who participated in one of our treatment programs supplemented their therapies by providing each other with support and encouragement. "Therapy gave us the initial push we needed," one recounted. The other explained how they finally overcame their fear of parties and dating: "We constantly pumped each other up, constantly telling each other that we could just do it."

HOW TO LOOK FOR A GOOD THERAPIST

You should consider getting an evaluation from a professional if your own efforts are not resulting in significant progress and social anxiety is limiting you or interfering with your happiness. One common source for finding a therapist is a friend or family member who may recommend someone he or she has seen and liked. This may be useful, but many people with social phobia will be uncomfortable about revealing their problem to friends or family. Also, a friend may have experienced a very different problem, and his or her therapist may not have expertise in social phobia.

It is desirable to find a therapist with particular expertise in treatment of anxiety problems. Mental health consumer organizations such as the Anxiety Disorders Association of America maintain referral lists of such experts, as do national and local professional associations and hospital-based referral services. Other sources include a family doctor or an HMO or other insurance program. A list of referral sources and their telephone numbers can be found in the appendix of this book. It is a good idea to obtain the names of several therapists and to conduct brief interviews on the telephone to help determine which one is right for you.

WHAT KIND OF THERAPIST?

Looking for the therapist you need in the mental health field can be very confusing. Therapists come in all shapes, sizes, and appellations. For example, the terms "therapist" and "psychotherapist" are quite broad and are often used by unlicensed therapists. Professional titles, such as "psychologist," "psychiatrist," and "social worker," however, are regulated in most states and can be used only by licensed professionals. So be sure to ask if the therapist is professionally licensed.

A therapist with a cognitive-behavioral approach will often be a psychologist with a Ph.D. (a doctoral degree from a university program in clinical psychology), although not all psychologists use such an approach. A therapist may also be a psychiatrist, who has an M.D. degree (is a doctor of medicine with specialty training in psychiatry). In addition to providing therapy, psychiatrists are licensed to prescribe medication. Other therapists include psychologists with degrees in education (Ed.D.) or in professional psychology (Psy.D.), and social workers with either a master's degree (M.S.W.) or a doctoral degree (D.S.W.) from a school of social work.

Regardless of the type of degree, important factors to consider are the therapist's knowledge of social anxiety and experience in treating this type of problem. One way to get this information is to ask the therapist directly: "What experience do you have in treating social phobia? What is your basic approach? What specific techniques do you use?" While it is a rare therapist whose area of specialty is social anxiety in particular, there are many therapists with sufficient experience in treating problems in the broader area of anxiety and phobias.

It is a good idea to consider in advance whether you have any preferences in regard to type of therapy. If you prefer a more direct treatment that targets changes in social behavior and anxiety as the primary goals, then seek out a therapist with a cognitive-behavioral approach. If you prefer a cognitive-behavioral group therapy, find out from consumer or professional organizations if it is available in your area. Other therapists use treatment approaches that are not cognitive or behavioral but may be highly effective. For example, if it is important to you to seek an understanding of life experiences that might have contributed to your anxiety problem, you will prefer to seek a more traditional insight-oriented type of therapy. For children, we recommend that parents seek out a therapist who can offer behavior therapy and who provides advice to parents as well as individual counseling for the child.

OTHER CONSIDERATIONS

In searching for a therapist, it is also important to acknowledge your personal preferences and to value your intuition. Have you been referred to a male therapist but would prefer a female therapist? Do you like the therapist? Does the therapist seem to understand your problem? There is solid research evidence that a "good match" between the patient's and therapist's values and personal style is important in determining the success of any therapy.

On the practical side, it is important to find out before your first visit whether the therapist will be able to provide treatment or merely an initial evaluation of your problem (usually followed by a referral to another therapist). It is important to ask if the therapist is able to schedule regular appointments at a convenient time. The therapist should tell you the fee and length of time for the initial session and for subsequent visits. Investing a bit of time doing a careful investigation before you begin therapy is usually well worth the effort.

MEDICATION TREATMENTS

The desire to be healed has always been part of health.

Seneca, 4 B.C.–A.D. 65

Why consider medication for social anxiety problems? As we have discussed, social phobia can cause a great deal of suffering. Psychotherapies can be helpful, but for some people they are only partially effective. And the biological roots and physical symptoms of social phobia suggest that treatments that address these factors could be useful.

Little was known about medication treatment for social phobia until the mid-1980s, long after medicines had been shown to be effective treatments for other emotional problems such as depression and panic attacks. In the past decade, study of medication treatments for social phobia has begun to catch up. This research has been stimulated by the growing recognition that social phobia is common, severe, and at least in part biologically based. Another factor has been the development of promising new antianxiety medications. Pharmaceutical manufacturers have recently taken notice of this work and recognized that persons with social phobia are potentially a large market for new medications that might prove helpful. They have jumped on the bandwagon and begun to invest resources into testing the effectiveness of their new medications for persons with social phobia.

The result of this new attention from academic psychiatrists and from drug companies is that controlled trials have shown that several medicines can alleviate the symptoms of social phobia, and these medicines are now moving into common use. This chapter will review the development of these medications, describe their benefits and limitations, and discuss some issues to consider in deciding whether to try a medication treatment for social phobia. Of course, any decision about whether to use a medication and the selection of an appropriate medication must be made in consultation with a physician who has confirmed the diagnosis and considered the medication's safety and benefits for an individual patient.

All of the medicines we will discuss have been evaluated in scientific studies of persons with social phobia, but each was initially approved to be marketed for another condition, such as depression or high blood pressure. In the United States, the Food and Drug Administration (FDA) has not yet approved any medication *specifically* for social phobia, although this will likely change in the next few years. Drugs the FDA has approved for one condition, however, are routinely later used by physicians for a variety of other conditions. Even when there is evidence that a drug that has been approved for one condition works for another condition (such as social phobia), manufacturers often decide not to pursue the lengthy and expensive application process the FDA requires before it will approve the drug specifically for the new condition.

BETA-BLOCKERS

Among the first medications to catch the attention of researchers interested in treatment of anxiety were the beta-adrenergic blockers, commonly known as beta-blockers. These were introduced in the 1960s as a new class of high blood pressure drugs, but beta-blockers have since been shown to have a number of other uses. Inderal (generic name propranolol) is the best known of these medications.

How They Work

The mechanism of these drugs made them intriguing to researchers who were interested in the treatment of anxiety problems. These medications are known as beta-blockers because they literally block the beta-receptors for the blood-borne hormone adrenaline. Beta-receptors are located in such organs as the heart and muscles. With a beta-blocker securely locking the adrenaline molecule out of its receptors, the hormone cannot trigger the symptoms it is known for, including a racing heart and trembling hands.

The normal role of adrenaline is to help activate the fight-or-flight response, which prepares a person to cope with mortal danger. If a person walks around a corner and is greeted by a lunging pit bull, a surge of adrenaline boosts the person's ability to either fight the attacker or escape by fleeing. For more ordinary "dangers," however, such as public speaking, performing onstage, or performing precision sports, the hormone's effects are sometimes more harmful than helpful. Fighting and fleeing are not desirable options in these situations. Here the effects of adrenaline contribute to the experience of performance anxiety, causing distressing symptoms that may lead to embarrassment and distract the person from the task at hand. Blocking the effects of adrenaline could prevent many of these performance anxiety symptoms.

Effectiveness

Sure enough, beta-blockers, taken in a single dose about one hour before a performance, have been shown to be effective treatments for anxiety in a variety of performance situations. They have been shown in research studies to benefit anxious musicians, bowlers, target shooters, and students with "examination nerves." Anxious performers taking beta-blockers tend to report that their usual physical symptoms are less intense and less distracting. In studies comparing the effects of beta-blockers with the effects of placebos (identical-looking but inactive pills) in anxious performers, judges (who are "blind" to what pill the performer is actually getting) generally report superior performance quality for performers taking the real medication.

Other recent studies have found that some beta-blockers are not very effective, however, when they are given on a daily basis to persons with generalized social phobia. These persons' fears encompass most social situations, not just performance situations. It is not clear if beta-blockers were less effective in these studies because they were given on a daily, as opposed to an intermittent, basis, or because they are less effective for anxiety in general social situations (such as making small talk with acquaintances) than they are for the anxiety that occurs in performance situations (such as public speaking). Fear of general social situations may be less likely to involve the adrenaline-based fight-or-flight response, which beta-blockers prevent. So beta-blockers appear to be most useful in social phobia for persons who need to take them only on an as-needed basis for performance anxiety.

There are many different beta-blockers on the market. They vary in several features, including their duration of action (from a few hours to about twenty-four hours). They also differ in the extent to which they affect two different types of beta-receptors, which are distributed on different organs of the body. Some beta-blockers mainly act on beta-1 receptors, where they can slow a racing heart, but they may have relatively little effect on relaxing shaky hands, which are controlled by beta-2 receptors in the muscles. Others, like Inderal, strongly affect both groups of beta-receptors. A typical dosage of Inderal for performance anxiety is 20 to 40 milligrams, taken about an hour before the performance.

Limitations

Besides the possible limitation of their benefit to situations involving performance anxiety, beta-blockers may also be less effective at reducing fearful thoughts than they are at reducing the physical symptoms of anxiety. People whose anxiety is made up of mainly fearful thoughts, with few accompanying physical arousal symptoms such as tremors, sweating, blushing, and palpitations, may be less likely to benefit from these medicines in their feared situations.

Taking beta-blockers on an as-needed basis can be convenient for occasional performance events, but it can be problematic when performances come up unexpectedly (such as being asked to make an impromptu presentation at a meeting) or when performance situations come up very frequently. When they are taken on a daily basis, beta-blockers may lose some effectiveness. Also, in performances that require great physical exertion (for example, tennis competitions), beta-blockers could limit peak athletic performance.

Beta-blockers also do not appear to be helpful in improving the performances of performers who are not particularly anxious to start with. For performers with only mild levels of anxiety, naturally occurring adrenaline is useful in contributing a sense of energy that gets channeled into focusing concentration and expressing emotions and even inspiration. If a person's naturally occurring level of nervous energy is already optimal for bringing out his or her best, using beta-blockers may actually detract from performance quality.

Side Effects

Beta-blockers generally need to be avoided in persons with asthma, diabetes, or certain forms of heart disease, so physicians often do an electrocardiogram (EKG) before starting treatment. In our experience, healthy persons usually experience minimal or no side effects with occasional use of beta-blockers. This is a major advantage of beta-blockers over other medications. Notably, they usually do not cause drowsiness and do not interfere significantly with mental sharpness or reaction time.

Beta-blockers are not physically addictive, and people do not crave or abuse them. It is important to recognize, however, that any medicine that quickly and reliably removes disturbing symptoms can create a psychological dependence. Performers may come to feel that they need to take a beta-blocker in order to go onstage. This sort of psychological dependence seems more likely to occur with medicines, such as beta-blockers, that are taken as needed directly before feared situations, as opposed to other types of medications such as SSRIs (see below), which are taken on a regular daily schedule.

Beta-Blockers Onstage

The widespread use of beta-blockers by musical performers has stirred some controversy. A 1987 survey of over two thousand members of the International Conference of Symphony and Opera Musicians found that 27 percent had used the beta-blocker propranolol for performance anxiety. Among this group of musicians who had used beta-blockers, 19 percent used prescribed beta-blockers daily, 11 percent used prescribed beta-blockers occasionally, and 70 percent reported obtaining these prescription drugs without any prescription for at least occasional use. Some persons in the musical community have criticized beta-blocker use by performers as excessive and inappropriate, a sign of personal and professional weakness. Others have defended it as a useful aid to survival in an intensely competitive field.

When a musician uses a beta-blocker to improve performance in a highly competitive audition for a symphony orchestra, is he or she essentially cheating? Is this situation the equivalent of an Olympic athlete's using steroids? Or is it no less fair than other acceptable uses of technology, such as purchasing better athletic shoes or a better-quality instrument to improve one's performance? Or is it instead simply a way for someone who has been disabled by an anxiety disorder to level the playing field, no more a form of cheating than allowing an athlete disabled by a painful knee injury to take aspirin?

We think it depends on the purpose for which the medication is being used. Unlike the use of steroids by an athlete to build extraordinary muscles, beta-blockers do not provide a musician with skills that are beyond his or her ordinary capabilities when relaxed, such as when practicing alone. While steroids can help any athlete grow muscles, beta-blockers do not improve performance for musicians who are not suffering from significant performance anxiety to start with. In this way beta-blockers function more like aspirin does as a pain reliever—they relieve the symptoms of a disorder.

So it seems misguided to argue that it is morally wrong for an anxious performer to use beta-blockers. Use of these anxiety-reducing medications, however, still may not be in the best interests of many performers. They certainly should not be used as a substitute for attempting to learn ways to master performance anxiety, especially for young performers. Even for persistent problems of experienced performers, nonmedication treatment alternatives such as cognitive-behavioral therapy should be considered first. These offer the greatest potential for long-term mastery over anxiety after treatment is discontinued.

Beta-blockers may be most helpful when used temporarily to allow a person to perform while he or she works on developing coping skills, in the same way a crutch allows a person to continue functioning while a broken leg heals. Despite their best efforts to cope, some performers will end up doing best with ongoing intermittent use of beta-blockers. Whether or not to use a beta-blocker should be a medically guided individual decision based on the severity of the performer's impairment and integrated into a long-term plan for managing the problem.

BENZODIAZEPINES

When people mention anti-anxiety drugs, they are usually referring to benzodiazepines. These are also known as minor tranquilizers, and

Valium (generic name diazepam) and Xanax (alprazolam) are among the best known. When these medications became available in the early 1960s, they were a major advance over older antianxiety drugs, because benzodiazepines are safer in general and much safer in overdose than older drugs such as barbiturates.

How They Work

Unlike beta-blockers, which act at beta-receptors located in a variety of organs throughout the body, these medications act on the anxiety signal at its origin in the brain, affecting a neurotransmitter called GABA (gamma aminobutyric acid). Benzodiazepines can work dramatically, often reducing anxiety symptoms within fifteen minutes. While they were initially found to relieve generalized anxiety (excessive tension and worrying), these medications have since been shown to work for other specific forms of anxiety as well, such as panic attacks.

Effectiveness

Because benzodiazepines work quickly, as do beta-blockers, there has been some testing of the effects of these medications when they are taken in a single dose before a performance situation, such as public speaking. Single doses of these drugs, taken on an as-needed basis, do reduce performance anxiety. Unfortunately, single doses also cause fatigue and drowsiness for some people, and they can take the edge off the mental sharpness or physical reaction time needed for an optimal performance.

Surprisingly, this problem is often sidestepped when benzodiazepines are taken on a regular schedule, two to four times per day. When a person takes these medicines regularly, the body adapts to them and side effects of fatigue and mental slowing usually diminish greatly. Fortunately, the antianxiety effects usually remain. Among the dozen or so benzodiazepines on the market, two have been studied specifically for social phobia—Xanax (alprazolam) and Klonopin (clonazepam). In the best-designed study to date, Klonopin or a dummy pill (placebo) was given on a regular schedule for twelve weeks to patients with social phobia (most of whom feared a variety of social situations, not just performing in public). Seventy-eight percent of the patients who were given Klonopin showed clear-cut improvement in anxiety symptoms and social functioning, compared to only about 20 percent of patients who were given the placebo. Further testing is needed to determine whether other benzodiazepines have similar benefits.

Limitations

Benzodiazepines have two major disadvantages. When they are taken daily, the body automatically develops a physical dependence on them. This means that a person planning to discontinue a benzodiazepine must do so gradually, usually over a period of at least several weeks. Stopping these medicines abruptly risks a rebound of anxiety and can cause withdrawal effects, including the rare occurrence of seizures.

Additionally, these medications have the potential to be abused. Excessive doses cause drowsiness, and benzodiazepines can be used to escape from real-world pressures and stop functioning, rather than to help cope with the same pressures and function better. People who have had problems with alcohol or drug abuse should generally avoid benzodiazepines because of this risk of abuse. For others, however, the risk of abusing these drugs in the course of supervised treatment for social phobia is very low. See opposite for more discussion of the controversy over benzodiazepine abuse.

Side Effects

Fatigue or drowsiness is by far the most common side effect of benzodiazepines, especially when they are first started and when the dose is being increased. Clumsiness or other problems with coordination can also occur. These effects tend to lessen or disappear after a few days of taking a regular dose of the medication. Alcohol taken in combination with benzodiazepines can have much stronger effects than usual and is potentially dangerous.

Most people taking these medicines on a regular basis have few ongoing side effects. Some that can occur are fatigue, sleeping longer, forgetfulness, impaired coordination, and loss of interest in sex. Benzodiazepines are not antidepressants, and they can occasionally worsen depression. Rarely, benzodiazepine treatment overshoots its goal and reduces a person's anxiety to less than a normal level, and the person may become too uninhibited—for example, expressing criticism he or she later regrets.

The Benzodiazepine Controversy

These drugs got a bad rep in the 1970s, when frequent prescribing of benzodiazepines for even mild forms of anxiety led to the widespread perception that much of America was "addicted" to Valium. Alarms were sounded in the media, and state governments responded with restrictions on the prescription of these drugs. Today, most physicians and their patients are appropriately concerned about the addictive potential of these medications. Unfortunately, some physicians have responded with a knee-jerk reaction, avoiding these useful medications at all costs.

It is important to weigh the real risks and benefits of these medications on a case-by-case basis. Our experience is that when these drugs are used under medical supervision for the treatment of social phobia, the risk of abuse is extremely low. This has been confirmed by larger studies of benzodiazepine use and abuse in the treatment of other anxiety problems. The risk of abuse is more considerable in persons who have previously abused alcohol or sedatives, or in persons currently abusing cocaine or other stimulant drugs, who may turn to benzodiazepines to come down from a nervous "high."

More common than abuse is the development of physical dependence, which needs to be considered when deciding whether to use benzodiazepines to treat social phobia. People taking benzodiazepines regularly do develop a physical dependence on the medicine, as do people who regularly take a high blood pressure medication. Stopping such medicines suddenly can be dangerous. Stopping benzodiazepines gradually is not dangerous, but it can lead to some temporary increase in anxiety. This "rebound anxiety" is most likely to occur around the time when the medicine is discontinued, although it is less common when the benzodiazepine dose has first been decreased very gradually over weeks. For these reasons, benzodiazepines are somewhat trickier to discontinue than other medications we discuss here, but for most people this difficulty consists of coping with a few days of somewhat increased anxiety.

SELECTIVE SEROTONIN REUPTAKE INHIBITORS (SSRIs)

These medications are the new kids on the antianxiety block. Introduced in the late 1980s as antidepressants, they have since been hailed as miracle drugs, unfairly vilified as murderers, researched like mad, and prescribed by the millions. The solid but unspectacular truth that has emerged from this confusion is that SSRIs are more effective than the older generation of antidepressants for some (but not all) conditions, and they have fewer side effects on the average. Prozac (generic name fluoxetine) was the first of the SSRIs to be marketed in the United States. Three others have since become available: Zoloft (sertraline), Paxil (paroxetine), and Luvox (fluvoxamine).

How They Work

Like most known antidepressants, the SSRIs work by blocking the uptake of particular chemical signaling agents (neurotransmitters) into nerve cells. In this way they regulate the activity of the neurotransmitter in the brain. Their benefits appear gradually, usually over a period of four to eight weeks. Unlike the older antidepressants, SSRIs are "cleaner" in that they mainly affect the neurotransmitter serotonin, with only minimal unwanted direct effects on other systems. For this reason they are relatively free of the annoying side effects—such as dry mouth, constipation, and drowsiness—that have limited the tolerability of older medications such as tricyclic antidepressants (TCAs). While initially marketed as a treatment for depression, SSRIs have been shown to be useful in a variety of conditions, including other anxiety disorders such as obsessive-compulsive disorder and panic disorder.

Effectiveness

Case reports in the medical literature of the effectiveness of SSRIs for social phobia have been building since these medicines were first introduced. In recent years there also have emerged placebo-controlled scientific studies that back up the initial findings. For each of the four SSRIs on the market in the United States (Prozac, Zoloft, Paxil, and Luvox), there is now some evidence for effectiveness in social phobia. An important difference from the benzodiazepines and the beta-blockers in the way these medicines can be used is that SSRIs are effective only when they are given on a daily basis for at least a few weeks. While the effects of SSRIs come on more gradually, they can be equally powerful.

Most studies of SSRIs for social phobia have found that 50 to 75 percent of patients show clear improvement in anxiety symptoms and social functioning after eight to twelve weeks of treatment. Most patients in these studies had been suffering from generalized fear of most social situations, but patients with anxiety limited to performance situations such as public speaking have been reported to benefit as well.

For people with some depression mixed in with social phobia, the antidepressant action of SSRIs offers an advantage over beta-blockers or benzodiazepines. (For people who have social phobia without depression, SSRIs typically help the social phobia without changing normal mood.) The main advantage of SSRIs for social phobia, however, does not lie in superior effectiveness compared to other effective treatments but rather in their relative freedom from side effects.

Limitations

Restrictions on the use of these medicines are relatively few. SSRIs do not cause much physical dependence, and because they are moderate- or long-acting they leave the body gradually, so discontinuation of SSRIs usually does not cause withdrawal effects. Taking higher than prescribed doses of SSRIs will not induce a "high" in any way, shape, or form, so abuse of these drugs is not a problem. These medications may even prove to be a helpful component of a treatment program for recovering substance abusers who have persistent social phobia. Because SSRIs have relatively little effect on other body systems, they are often safer than other medications for people with medical problems, such as heart conditions.

Persons taking SSRIs do need to be aware that these medicines can interact with many other prescription and over-the-counter medications. This may require dosage adjustments of the other medication, so the safety of taking any medicine in combination with SSRIs should be checked with a physician.

Side Effects

While an advantage of the SSRIs is that most people experience few side effects from them, they do cause annoying or intolerable side effects for some people. Among the most common side effects are restless sleep (often accompanied by increased recall of dreams) and some loss of appetite or nausea, which usually disappears in a few days. Fatigue and increased sweating are occasionally problems.

Sexual side effects such as decreased interest and delay or difficulty in reaching orgasm affect a proportion of patients of both sexes.

People who, in addition to having social phobia, are prone to unexpected panic attacks (severe anxiety attacks that are not related to social fears or social situations) may be particularly sensitive to these medicines. Extra-low starting doses may be desirable for such people to avoid an initial temporary worsening of anxiety symptoms. Early claims in the media that Prozac treatment caused an increased risk of suicidal or homicidal behavior have not held up in systematic studies of the rates of such behavior among thousands of people taking Prozac.

Does Prozac Change Personality?

Psychiatrist Peter Kramer, in his book *Listening to Prozac,* has raised the controversial issue of whether Prozac and medications like it can change personality. Kramer never actually uses the term "social phobia" in his book. In many of the cases he uses to illustrate personality change, however, some of the key effects of Prozac are relief of social phobic inhibitions. He describes the case of Tess, for example, whom he had recently started on Prozac:

> I have never seen a patient's social life reshaped so rapidly and dramatically. Low self-worth, competitiveness, jealousy, poor interpersonal skills, shyness, fear of intimacy—the usual causes of social awkwardness—are so deeply ingrained and so difficult to influence that ordinarily change comes gradually if at all. But Tess blossomed all at once. . . . I believe Tess's story contains an unchronicled reason for Prozac's enormous popularity: its ability to alter personality. Here was a patient whose usual method of functioning changed dramatically. She became socially capable, no longer a wallflower but a social butterfly.

Social phobia, and the way it can improve with medication treatment, does challenge our notions of what really makes up a personality. If the easing of lifelong social inhibitions can be called a change in personality, there is little doubt that SSRIs and other medications can sometimes have such effect. Outside observers, who never knew the inner experience of Tess,

may have inferred from her more assertive and outgoing behavior that her personality had actually changed. It is quite
rare, however, for a person who experiences relief from social
anxiety and avoidance while taking an SSRI to consider this to
be a personality change. More commonly, patients like Tess
experience the change as an ability to more fully express their
true personalities, the spontaneous thoughts and feelings that
had been kept bottled up by fear.

For persons who are about to start treatment for lifelong
problems of being easily embarrassed and avoiding social opportunities, it may be impossible to imagine life without these
familiar burdens. When change then comes rapidly, as it sometimes does with medication, it can be confusing, even if it is
welcome. Occasionally a patient does question whether his or
her personality has changed.

At age thirty-two, a lifetime of painful shyness had left Elaine
feeling at a loss. Having recently ended a disappointing relationship with a boyfriend, she knew it would be agony to
reenter the party circuit and try to meet someone new. In the
past, she tended to settle for the first decent guy who showed
interest in her, but she knew she deserved better. She would
rationalize her shyness by telling herself that any woman who
pursued a man was just behaving out of desperation, which
was beneath her dignity. Rather than confronting her social
fears, which seemed insurmountable to Elaine, she coped by
persuading herself that her real problem was the insensitivity
of men. If only the guy at work she secretly admired were
sensitive enough to read her mind . . .

Elaine decided to take what felt like a desperate chance. She
called a local clinic that had advertised its research studies on
social phobia, and although skeptical she gave Prozac a try.
During the third week of treatment, something happened that
seemed strange to her. She started a conversation with the
guy she had admired at work and actually enjoyed it. While
speaking, she even looked him in the eye—a rarity for her.
Soon it became a rarity no longer. She found herself relishing
ordinary contact with people in a way she never had before.
On the one hand, it was delightful, but on the other, it was
confusing. As she put it, "Is this the real Elaine, or is it Prozac-
talking?" The strangeness of her behavior bothered her to

the point that she even considered stopping the medication.

As we began to explore just who she really was, it became clearer to Elaine that Prozac had not changed her fundamental identity. But as she acknowledged this, she had to confront the painful truth that many of her cherished beliefs about the flaws of people around her had been products of her defensiveness over her own limitations. Now that she was less limited socially, Elaine could recognize that being outgoing wasn't desperate behavior, as she had once labeled it in others. She began to conclude that men were only relatively insensitive. Elaine resisted her first inclination to reject the medication and the unfamiliar feelings it had brought, and she decided to rethink some of her faulty assumptions about people instead.

After a year of combined medication and psychotherapy treatment, during which her early improvement continued and progressed, we decided to try discontinuing the medication. At this point Elaine wasn't sure if her new social ease depended on continuing the Prozac or if it could be sustained as a result of the many positive experiences she'd had in the last year. After stopping the medicine for a few months, Elaine found that some of her fears of people had crept back, but she was successfully fighting them instead of giving in to them. Although grateful for the boost Prozac had given her, she felt no need or desire to resume taking it.

MONOAMINE OXIDASE INHIBITORS (MAOIs)

MAOIs are the medications that first made psychiatric researchers stand up and take notice of the potential of medication to benefit persons with social phobia. Since the late 1950s, MAOIs had been known to be effective antidepressants. In Britain, several studies in the 1960s showed that MAOIs were helpful for phobias in general, but researchers had not focused on social phobia in particular. They also noted that among other patients who had major depression, an atypical subgroup with emotional overreactivity responded better to MAOIs than to other antidepressants.

Meanwhile, in New York, psychiatrist Donald Klein had been studying a group of patients he called "hysteroid dysphoric," who were difficult to treat by the standard psychoanalytic methods of the time. Klein, a leading innovator in the then-young field of psychopharmacology, conceptualized the key feature of these patients as a biologically based extreme sensitivity to rejection. In these patients, the end of a brief love affair might lead to desperate unhappiness and taking to bed for days. He demonstrated that these patients, too, benefited markedly from MAOIs. During treatment, they no longer experienced every rejection as a devastating loss.

In the early 1980s, psychiatrist Michael Liebowitz was studying panic attacks and agoraphobia with the New York State Psychiatric Institute team led by Klein. The researchers were puzzled by a patient with panic disorder and agoraphobia who didn't do well with imipramine, which was the highly effective standard medication treatment for panic disorder at the time. The patient's main complaint was feeling panicky on trains, a common problem among persons with agoraphobia, who tend to fear that if they have a frightening panic attack on a train they will be unable to escape or get help.

In reviewing this patient's symptoms, the researchers began to suspect that the patient had been misdiagnosed. His panicky feelings on the train were not due to the usual fear of being unable to get help. Instead, he most feared that other passengers would notice his anxiety and that he would feel humiliated. When a train was empty, he was completely relieved, whereas a true agoraphobic would feel more frightened than ever if left alone in that situation. The patient actually had social phobia, and it turned out that he eventually responded remarkably well to the MAOI called Nardil (generic name phenelzine).

Liebowitz recognized the thread of interpersonal hypersensitivity and MAOI responsiveness that ran through atypical depression, hysteroid dysphoria, and now social phobia. Whereas social phobia was previously thought to be uncommon, once Liebowitz had scratched the surface of recognizing social phobia and had begun actively to seek out more patients for research, volunteers with social phobia started coming out in droves. He became aware that social phobia was far more common and devastating than generally was believed at the time. Liebowitz called on psychiatrists to reconsider this "neglected anxiety disorder" from a biological perspective. He showed in a placebo-controlled study that MAOIs were highly effective for social phobia, a finding that has since been confirmed by other research groups in the United States and around the world.

How They Work

MAOIs work by inhibiting the activity of a particular enzyme, monoamine oxidase (MAO), which is an important regulator of several neurotransmitters in the brain. There are currently two MAOIs on the market in the United States, Nardil (phenelzine) and Parnate (tranylcypromine).

Effectiveness

The MAOI Nardil is currently the best-established medication treatment for social phobia, and it also may be the medication with the most powerful effects on social phobia. In well-designed, placebo-controlled studies at several independent research centers, Nardil has consistently benefited two thirds or more of social phobia patients who have taken it over an eight- to twelve-week study. Even more so than for the SSRIs, when Nardil is effective, the results can be dramatic. Also, when other medications fail to help, MAOIs sometimes work better. As is true for other antidepressants, the benefits of MAOIs usually take at least a few weeks to begin to show.

Limitations

Unfortunately, MAOIs also have serious limitations. Of greatest concern is the so-called cheese reaction. Certain foods, including most aged cheeses, need to be avoided by patients taking MAOIs, because the foods can interact with MAOIs to cause a sudden rise in blood pressure and such symptoms as headache and vomiting. If a severe high blood pressure reaction occurs and is not promptly treated, it has the potential to cause a stroke or even death.

For this reason, patients taking MAOIs need to follow a strict diet avoiding the dangerous foods, which include many aged foods (such as sausages), most alcoholic beverages, and an assortment of other oddities such as marmite and fava beans. Certain prescription and over-the-counter medications, such as decongestants, are also strictly prohibited. Despite this frightening risk, most patients can follow the restrictions without major inconvenience, and even mild high blood pressure reactions are uncommon occurrences.

Side Effects

Whereas the cheese reaction poses a serious risk but is uncommon when precautions are taken, other MAOI side effects occur commonly but are rarely dangerous. One frequently troubling problem is fatigue or drowsiness, especially in the mid-afternoon. Others that sometimes occur include light-headedness (especially when suddenly standing up), sexual functioning difficulties, and weight gain. Some of these side effects wane in intensity as a person adjusts to the medicine over a period of several weeks. The fact that well-informed patients commonly take these difficult medications despite the above concerns, and do well with them, is a testament to the powerful effectiveness of MAOIs against the symptoms of social phobia.

MAOIs: THE NEXT GENERATION

The frustrating combination of high effectiveness but relatively high risk of side effects for MAOIs has spurred research into drugs that might combine their benefits with greater safety and comfort. RIMAs just might fit the bill. RIMAs, or reversible inhibitors of monoamine oxidase, inhibit the same enzyme as MAOIs but do so less completely. The implications of this are that RIMAs are far safer than the standard MAOIs and have fewer annoying side effects as well. Moclobemide, a RIMA that is currently marketed in Canada, Europe, and much of the world outside the United States, has been used safely without stringent dietary restrictions.

If this sounds too good to be true, however, it may be. While moclobemide looked almost as effective as Nardil for social phobia in one study, a more recent study, conducted by one of us (F.S.), suggested that its benefits may be considerably less impressive. Moclobemide is being marketed for social phobia in some Europeon countries, but it is not expected to become available in the U.S. anytime soon. Meanwhile, research continues on other newer medicines in this promising class.

Should Everyone Be On Prozac?

Just as the discovery by anxious musicians of beta-blockers in the 1970s led to concerns about unfair advantage and overuse, the development and growing acceptance of medication treatment for generalized social phobia in the 1990s has raised similar controversy. If drugs such as Prozac and Paxil can turn a wallflower into a social butterfly, what can they do for those of us who are just occasionally troubled by self-consciousness or shyness? And we are not talking about just a few million people: Surveys suggest that most college students report feeling embarrassment at least once a week, and younger teenagers get embarrassed even more often. Wouldn't any moder-

234 TREATMENT FOR SOCIAL PHOBIA

ately successful businessman really like to become an "alpha male," rising to the top of the corporate hierarchy like the medicated monkeys in Raleigh's study (as we discussed in chapter 9)?

While the vision of every man a Donald Trump, every woman a Madonna is certainly chilling (although Madonna, too, has acknowledged suffering performance anxiety), these notions are based on a few dubious premises.

The first misconception is that if these medications help patients with social phobia become more comfortable and assertive, they must cause people with only mild shyness or embarrassment to become "supersociable" and aggressive. With rare exception, this is not the case. When nondepressed people take antidepressants, studies show that they mostly just remain nondepressed and do not become "superhappy." There is no evidence to suggest that people with mild social reticence become party animals when taking SSRIs, benzodiazepines, or MAOIs, or that moderately successful businessmen become CEOs of Fortune 500 companies, or that decent public speakers become mesmerizing orators.

Second, while there will always be some people eager to try anything to "perfect" themselves if they believe it will be effortless, it seems unlikely that most people with trivial social anxiety would be willing to seek out a doctor who will prescribe indiscriminately, willing to spend $100 a month or more on the latest medications plus doctor's fees for monitoring the treatment over an indefinite period, willing to run the risk of annoying side effects such as restless sleep and sexual difficulties, and willing to accept the unknown risks inherent in long-term use of any medication.

In our experience, most patients turn to medication treatment only after years of suffering, failure of self-help and psychotherapy approaches, and a great deal of soul-searching. They debate the pros and cons of taking a medicine, even a beneficial and safe medicine, that might affect the way they think or behave. Studies of doctors' prescribing patterns for treatment of emotional conditions have consistently shown underprescribing, even for severe disorders such as major depression that are well-known to respond to medication. Only a fraction of persons with objective mental illness now get even merely adequate medication treatment.

A third mistaken premise is that even if a medicine could

routinely render people completely free of social fears and inhibitions (which current medications cannot), such a state would be normal or at all desirable. If such freedom were obtainable from a medication, it would likely come as part of a package deal—along with freedom from sensitivity to others' needs, freedom from following norms for socially acceptable behavior, and perhaps freedom from following unpleasant laws. People have long been able to achieve such freedoms with high doses of alcohol, cocaine, or other easily available substances. Even if future miracle drugs could achieve these freer-than-normal states without the druggy "high" associated with drugs of abuse, the end result would more likely be an irritating, sociopathic social outcast rather than a supersocializer or a superbusinessman. These are not the results we see with today's medication treatments, which tend only to lessen severe social anxiety into something more manageable.

A Summary of Medications Used for Social Phobia

	Usual effectiveness	Severity of common side effects	Can take intermittently	Abuse potential	Antidepressant effects
Beta-blockers (e.g., Inderal)	+++[1]	-	yes	no	no
Benzodiazepines (e.g., Klonopin)	+++	--	yes	yes	no
SSRIs (e.g., Prozac)	+++	--	no	no	yes
MAOIS (e.g., Nardil)	++++	---	no	no	yes

Some other medicines that may be effective but need more study include: Buspar (buspirone), Effexor (venlafaxine), Anafranil (clomipramine), Welbutrin (bupropion), and Moclobemide[2]

Key: + fair; ++ good; +++ very good; ++++ most effective
 - very mild; -- mild; --- moderate

---

[1] But effect may be limited to anxiety related to performance situations.

[2] Moclobemide is not currently marketed in the United States.

ANSWERS TO SOME COMMON QUESTIONS ABOUT MEDICATION FOR SOCIAL PHOBIA

Q: *How severe must my social phobia be for me to consider medication?*

A: There is a common misconception that medication works only for the most severe cases of an emotional problem such as social phobia (perhaps only for hermits or very shy folks such as Frankenstein). In fact, medicines, like therapy, seem to work equally well (or even better) for milder cases of social phobia. Remember, by definition, even people with mild cases of social phobia are still experiencing social fear and/or avoidance that causes them a great deal of distress or interferes in a significant way with their ability to function at their best in social, school, or work situations. Both published research and our experience suggest that many, many more people who could benefit from medication either never seek help or suffer much too long before finally seeking help.

Q: *Isn't resorting to medicine a sign of failure or weakness?*

A: Most people do not take medication lightly, especially when it comes to taking it for emotional problems, and they shouldn't take it lightly. Not everyone who experiences social phobia wants or needs to seek medication treatment. But acknowledging a problem doesn't make it worse, and being able to take action to solve it is a sign of strength, not weakness. It is important to use medication to supplement but not to replace your own efforts to resolve problems. If you are making progress, neither you nor others will see you as a failure. Of course, people with social phobia are especially likely to worry about what others might think, including what they might think of their taking medication.

Q: *Do medicines cure social phobia, or do people need to stay on them indefinitely to stay well?*

A: Medicines are not a cure for social phobia, yet most people use medicines temporarily, typically for six to twelve months. The ideal length of treatment is not known.

In considering how medicines help treat social phobia, it is useful to remember that the problem has both biological and psychological elements. Depending on your symptoms, it may be most accurate to think of the biological part as an inborn tendency toward shyness and self-consciousness and/or a kind of physiological overreactivity—a tendency to blush, tremble, sweat, or get palpitations easily. The direct effects of medication for social phobia are to decrease these unwanted tendencies. These direct effects are present only while the medicine is in your system.

Relief of these biologically based tendencies also has indirect effects, however, on the psychological side of social phobia. When a medicine reduces self-consciousness or physical symptoms, it frees a person to think and behave differently, to change old unhelpful thought patterns and habits that have been learned over the years. These secondary changes sometimes outlast the direct effects of the medication.

Elaine, for example, was used to feeling shy, suppressing her desire to approach a man she liked, blaming the man for not reaching out to her, and thinking she was unattractive. Medication seemed to directly lessen her shyness and allowed her to be more outgoing. This led to new results that did not fit the old pattern she had learned: When she was outgoing she felt better about herself, and men were more interested in her. Over months of these positive experiences, she gradually "unlearned" old assumptions that she was unattractive and helpless, and discovered that being proactive led to better results. When she discontinued medication after a year of treatment, she noticed some increase in her tendency toward shyness. Her new attitudes didn't change, however, and she recognized that she could overcome her shyness by confronting it instead of giving in to it.

Elaine's experience was fairly typical. After a period of gaining confidence and unlearning old fears while on medication, upon stopping the medication symptoms typically partially return. Some people are able to maintain or surpass the level of improvement they had on the medicine. Others slip all the way back to where they started before medication. In the latter case, they may choose to resume the medicine for a longer period of time or to add some psychotherapy with the goal of reaching a more lasting improvement.

Q: *What are the long-term risks of being on these medicines?*

A: The classes of medicines in common use for social phobia have been marketed for anywhere from about seven to thirty-five years, so our knowledge varies depending on the medicine. Most of these medications have been taken by some people for as long as the medications have been available. Long-term use of these medicines has not been proven to be associated with serious health problems. Nevertheless, it makes sense to use any of these medicines for the minimum period of time needed. One approach is to try to discontinue treatment either after six to twelve months or after improvement has leveled off, whichever comes later. The optimal length of treatment may vary greatly from person to person.

Q: *If medication works for my social phobia, does it mean that I have a chemical imbalance in my brain?*

A: The term "chemical imbalance" is problematic. For one thing, it has always sounded too much to us like being "unbalanced," which Webster's defines as "deranged." Semantics and Freudian slips of the tongue aside, it seems that when it comes to the brain, response to a particular form of treatment, such as medicine or psychotherapy, tells us little about what caused the problem. For example, a recent brain-imaging study in patients with obsessive-compulsive disorder showed that two very different kinds of treatment, medication treatment and behavior therapy, induce the same changes in regional brain activity when they are effective. Whether social phobia is caused by life events, by genetics, or by a combination of the two, it is likely reflected in a person's brain chemistry in some way, although our current technology is not able to detect such differences meaningfully in individual patients.

Q: *What are the risks of these medications during pregnancy?*

A: Because the risks of taking these medicines during pregnancy or while breast-feeding are not completely known, it is important for women to avoid these medications during these times. Women of childbearing age should practice a reliable form of contraception before and during use of these medications. When pregnancy has occurred unexpectedly in a woman taking one of these medications, however, the risk of harm to the fetus generally appears to be low. Medication should usually be gradually discontinued at this point in consultation with a physician. Men taking these medications are not at increased risk for having children with birth defects.

Q: *Should I consider medicine, therapy, or both for my social phobia?*

A: The limited data we have comparing treatments suggests that the best medicine and therapy treatments for social phobia are roughly equally effective. Medications may work more quickly and may effect more dramatic improvement, but therapies may have more staying power after treatment is completed. At present, though, we don't have any hard facts on how to predict who will do best with a particular approach. Studies comparing medication and therapy treatments are currently under way and may clarify this in the future. Patients often have a strong gut feeling on this issue, and they often seek treatment of the particular type they prefer. Our thoughts are as follows:

For most people, trying a short-term psychological therapy alone is the most sensible first step in treatment of uncomplicated social phobia. Therapy has several obvious advantages. The very process of therapy demands a self-reliance that often makes success particularly fulfilling. Progress that is hard-won and due primarily to one's own efforts can build greater self-confidence than a technological solution such as medication. The evidence that short-term cognitive-behavioral therapy can produce long-term gains is another good reason to choose this approach.

After several months of good effort at a cognitive-behavioral approach, a reassessment is useful. If some progress has occurred, it may be worth giving the therapy more time or adding medication treatment to it. If no progress has occurred, or if fears have made it impossible to do the social exposure homework of cognitive-behavioral therapy, it is reasonable to consider medication. Alternatively, if deeper psychological issues have emerged as roadblocks, a more insight-oriented psychodynamic approach to therapy might be considered.

There are several circumstances in which medication is the clear first-choice treatment. One of these is the presence of substantial depression, which may make it impossible for a person to actively participate in psychotherapy. Another is when an extremely feared situation happens rarely—for example, a one-shot deal such as having to accept a retirement award onstage. In this case a person may prefer to seek the easiest short-term solution, which may be a single dose of medication.

Another possible circumstance in which medication is the first-choice treatment is when social phobia is severe. For such people, attempting psychotherapy may feel like paddling against a biological riptide. When social phobia is severe, medication may have some advantage over therapy.

Combined medication and cognitive-behavioral treatment works best for some people, and it may have synergistic effects. The medication can reduce fears to the point where people can progress faster in confronting their feared situations. The therapy can use psychological means to solidify these gains, so that they are less likely to fade away when the medication is discontinued.

Q: *How do I find a physician for medication treatment of social phobia?*

A: New information about social phobia and its treatment has been increasingly available to physicians, but patients cannot just assume that a doctor or even a psychiatrist is up-to-date in this area. If you already have a psychiatrist, it is perfectly acceptable to ask if he or she is knowledgeable about social phobia. If not, a consultation with an expert can be very helpful. See the appendix for organizations that can make referrals to specialists in social phobia.

Q: *Should children with social phobia ever take medication?*

A: There is a small but growing body of evidence that children with severe social phobia benefit from the same medications that help adults with social phobia. Selective mutism is a condition in which a child will not speak at all outside of the immediate family, often due to extreme shyness. These children may be very difficult for a therapist to "reach." In a controlled study of children with selective mutism, twelve weeks of treatment with Prozac was somewhat helpful and had only minimal side effects. It is possible that such medical intervention for selective mutism could stave off even more damaging emotional problems from developing and persisting in these children.

For children with the mildest forms of social anxiety, however, resorting to medication treatment sends a child the wrong message— that the problem is very serious and that medicines are the first way to solve social problems. The answer is less clear in children with social phobia of moderate severity that may be interfering with class- room performance and blocking the development of friendships and social skills. Certainly psychotherapy approaches should be tried first, and the threshold for trying a medication approach in children should be higher than that for adults. The safety of these medications in children has not been established as conclusively as it has been for adults. But if therapy is not working for a child, it does not mean that nothing else should be considered. There has been a disturbing tendency for adults, including health professionals, throughout history to ignore suffering in children that they would not tolerate in adults. If other approaches have failed, and if social phobia is seriously affect- ing a child's ability to function, short-term medication treatment might put a child back on track to normal social development. This is an area where more research is much needed.

20

THE FUTURE

As for the future, your task is not to foresee, but to enable it.

Antoine de Saint-Exupéry, 1948

For people with social anxiety or social phobia, the future is looking brighter. Over the past ten years these problems have received increasing attention from researchers and mental health professionals. With wider recognition of the disorder of social phobia, more people are learning that it is possible to help themselves and to be helped. New and more effective treatment approaches are being applied more widely. More people are availing themselves of treatment and learning to overcome their fears.

QUESTIONS REMAIN

Many questions remain to be answered, however, through research studies and treatment experience. Our treatments for social phobia are far from perfect—they usually help, but as is true for the treatment of most chronic problems from depression to diabetes, they rarely cure. We also have much to learn about predicting which particular type of treatment will offer the most benefit to a particular individual. It might turn out that public speaking phobias do best in group therapy, for example, or that persons who are most troubled by trembling do best with a particular medication. If we could determine a specific behavior, symptom pattern, or blood hormone level that predicted how

241

a person would respond to behavior therapy or to a particular medication, we would be able to select the most effective treatment from the very start. The treatment process could become more efficient and less expensive.

We also do not know the ideal length of treatment. While our short-term treatments produce good short-term results, the long-term results are not as well studied. The problem is that while social phobia tends to be a lifelong problem, most treatments have been studied over only weeks to months. Recent research suggests that cognitive-behavioral therapy is especially effective at producing long-term improvement, perhaps because it teaches coping techniques that individuals can continue to use long after the formal therapy has ended. It is important to understand why some people maintain improvement after a relatively short course of medication treatment, while others slip back. Although long-term studies tend to be more expensive and difficult to perform, we need to know more about how people do over the long haul—months and years after short-term treatment itself is completed.

Most efforts at treatment have focused on the segment of the population that suffers the most distress and impairment from social phobia—young adults. Although young adults are the age group most likely to seek treatment, often they have delayed seeking help for social anxiety for a decade or more, until they cannot bear it any longer. We would like to understand better how social phobia begins and what enables most toddlers and adolescents to overcome normal social fears on their own.

Learning how to identify children who are at high risk to develop social phobia may create opportunities for us to prevent social phobia. Parents, teachers, and pediatricians could be educated to identify such children and to modify their approaches to these kids in a way that will be beneficial. Wider dissemination of self-help approaches to teenagers and adults coping with social anxieties may be another way to prevent these fears from developing into more severe phobias. Prevention holds the potential for saving a great deal of human suffering, and it may also be a less costly alternative to treating serious problems later on.

Much of the genetic and biological underpinnings of social phobia also remains mysterious. We have clues that just might lead to powerful new ways to diagnose and treat this problem. New technologies are emerging and being refined, such as brain imaging, and these promise to revolutionize our understanding of the function and dysfunction of the brain. Promising new medications, such as the reversible MAOIs, need to be further tested to establish their benefits and safety in the treatment of social phobia.

SOCIETY'S CHOICES

Whether our society has the will to provide resources to help improve the prevention and treatment of social anxiety problems is another question, however. The stigma around mental disorders is still extremely pervasive, and in the absence of vocal advocacy for attention to these problems, mental health problems tend to get ignored. At a time when governments are cutting back their overall spending—and their spending for health care research in general—mental health care research is particularly vulnerable. Despite the tremendous strides in recognizing the devastating public health impact of severe social phobia, it remains widely underestimated and misunderstood, even among mental health professionals.

Unlike other physical disorders, and even some other mental disorders, social phobia has lacked an organized constituency of people who are willing to fight for attention to this problem. Perhaps this is a natural consequence of the difficulties with assertiveness and speaking out that plague people with social phobia, but it need not remain so. More broadly based mental health organizations, such as the Anxiety Disorders Association of America and Freedom From Fear, have stepped up to lead advocacy efforts to recognize social phobia along with other anxiety problems, such as panic disorder and obsessive-compulsive disorder. If the progress of recent years is to continue, advocates for the treatment of social anxiety problems will need to continue to organize better to press government, private foundations, and universities to devote appropriate resources to these problems.

The pharmaceutical industry, which has brought its economic might to bear in publicizing the diagnosis and treatment of those conditions for which it has developed medications, has only recently begun to turn its attention to social phobia. Much of the early research into medications for social phobia in the United States was done at medical schools by psychiatrists funded by the National Institute of Mental Health. Now that the pharmaceutical industry stands poised to profit from the new "market" for its products that persons with social phobia represent, it bears the responsibility of directing some of those profits toward helping persons with this disorder.

The goal of helping people recognize a treatable problem is in the common interest of both the industry and the general public. The pharmaceutical industry is in a position to play a humanitarian role in both educating people about the nature of these problems and supporting the work of scientists researching them. As pharmaceutical companies begin the process of seeking approval from drug regulatory agencies in some countries in order to market their drugs for treatment of social phobia, some industry resources are starting to flow in the direction of social phobia research and education.

A risk of pharmaceutical industry promotion of awareness of a condition and its treatments is that the industry may tend to underplay less profitable medications or alternative nonmedication approaches such as cognitive-behavioral therapy. Insurance companies and managed-care organizations similarly may exert inappropriate pressure to apply the cheapest and briefest treatments available. Such strategies will ultimately backfire, however, if patients are dissatisfied with the ineffective treatment they receive and if the companies end up spending more resources when partially treated problems worsen or recur. Recent pharmaceutical marketing campaigns for other mental disorders, such as obsessive-compulsive disorder, have recognized that spreading information about all treatment approaches tends to be good public relations. Enlightened self-interest has worked, on the whole, to benefit the public in this area.

THE RISKS OF KNOWLEDGE

The recognition and treatment of social phobia also carry some risks, as do the new treatment technologies. A basic question is whether all social anxiety problems need to be treated. Whereas few people would argue against providing help to a person who is so fearful of others that he or she is unable to work or to attend any social activities, what about someone with a milder case? At the mild end of the spectrum, social phobic problems merge with the everyday anxieties of normal social life. If we advocate the recognition and treatment of social phobia, are we inadvertently pathologizing the blushing bride, the nervous bar mitzvah boy, and the shy toddler?

It seems unlikely that treatments for social phobia will be widely overused by people who are not in serious emotional pain. In chapter 19 we discussed the concern that drugs such as Prozac might be used as "cosmetics" to flesh out the minor wrinkles in people's personalities. Our most effective treatments for social phobia, however, are not as easy to take as the media has suggested. Even the newest breakthrough medicines frequently have annoying side effects, are only partially effective, and can be quite expensive. Our most powerful psychological therapies require a substantial effort and a willingness to accept some anxiety and some risks of embarrassment in the service of overcoming more painful problems in the long run. These are not efforts to be taken lightly. As it now stands, only a tiny percentage of persons with clinical social phobia even seek treatment at all.

Whereas people with severe social phobia continue to be very much undertreated, people with very mild social anxiety, which causes only minor distress and no impairment, are best off simply learning to accept their sensitivity in this area. A substantial threat to such self-acceptance is the growing pressure in Western societies to attain un-achievable ideals of social behavior. Technology and the media have brought to every hamlet the images of superficial social perfection in appearance, in public speaking, and in social graces. More and more we live in a virtual reality of perfect images that are unreal—or at least not realistically attainable for most people. The social pres-sures to ''perform'' can be overwhelming.

In such an environment, is the cultivation of real but imperfect relationships in danger of becoming a lost art—just another cottage industry threatened by the assembly line? Or will the computer-driven global village of the future instead be a place where technology will bring diverse people closer together, fostering a new social tolerance; a place free of the social pressures that were a burden in the hierarchi-cal and socially unforgiving village life of the past?

CYBERSOCIETY

Computer society has classically held an allure for the socially awk-ward ''nerd'' as a place where ideas carry more weight than appear-ances and social graces. As cyberspace, with its own social etiquette, becomes a more and more important site for interpersonal dealings, will society's values be transformed in a similar direction? Will tradi-tional social skills lose some of their importance?

Today people can have ongoing relationships, even virtual sex, with people they know only through words and images they choose to send to a computer screen. Personal appearance and public speaking style are irrelevant to these relationships. Might a true ''revenge of the nerds'' transform society by deemphasizing appearance, social skills, and performance? It seems more likely instead that society at large will transform cyberspace gradually to foster prevailing social values and trends.

Microsoft chairman Bill Gates sees technology as a largely benign means of bringing people together. In his book *The Road Ahead,* he tells the story of a relationship he had that was maintained largely through electronic mail with a woman in another city. He describes how they were able to "sort of" see a movie together by planning over their cellular phones to see the same movie simultaneously in their respective cities, then discussing the movie afterward on those same cellular phones. He doesn't report the woman's opinion of this rather unromantic electronic "date," although he does promise that virtual dating will be better in the future because movie watching could be combined with a video conference!

We have already seen the first backlash to the aura of a virtual social life. Critics of the cyberspace community, such as Steve Jones, author of *Cybersociety,* contend that on-line communities lack a sense of commitment and a knowledge of other people, and that they will never replace real-life communities. There is a risk that people with social anxiety problems will use cyberspace as an escape from having to learn social skills, settling for virtual relationships over less controllable but ultimately more satisfying real ones.

On the other hand, visiting cyberspace in moderation holds promise for helping people get over their social fears. The anonymity of cyberspace discussion groups may provide a level of emotional safety that allows socially anxious people to start to speak up, try out their ideas on others, and get the kind of positive feedback that builds confidence, as occurs in a psychotherapy group. In this way, exposure to social cyberspace might serve as a confidence-building transition to trying out new real social situations.

Similarly, virtual reality simulators, which have already been applied to helping acrophobics overcome their fear of heights, might have a role in treating social phobia. They could be developed for persons with social phobia to simulate feared social situations, such as giving a speech to an audience. Depending on the severity of the patient's fears, the simulator could be set on different levels of audience size, and the audience's reactions could be preset for anything from constant applause and standing ovations to blank expressions or even a few yawns. Just how easily social confidence built in virtual reality or cyberspace can be transferred to real performances and relationships remains to be seen, however.

Regardless of what the future may hold, the progress that has been made in understanding social anxiety is real. We see it in the statistical results of our studies of diagnosing and treating social phobia and, most important, in the human responses of our patients. The challenges of combating old stigmas against emotional problems and coping with new pressures of modern society are daunting, and many questions remain to be answered. Whichever way society evolves, however, there is a new base of knowledge that we can use to relieve the suffering caused by this most human of all fears.

APPENDIX:
WHERE TO FIND HELP

The following professional and consumer organizations offer information and help with referrals for persons with social phobia or related conditions:

Professional Organizations
American Psychological
  Association
750 First Street, N.W.
Washington, DC 20002-4242
(202) 336-5800

American Psychiatric
  Association
1400 K Street, N.W.
Washington, DC 20005
(202) 682-6220

Association for the Advancement of Behavior Therapy
305 Seventh Avenue, Suite 16A
New York, NY 10001
(212) 647-1890

National Association of Social
  Workers
750 First Street, N.E.
Washington, DC 20002
(800) 638-8799

American Psychiatric Nurses
  Association
1200 Nineteenth Street, N.W.
Suite 300
Washington, DC 20036
(202) 857-1133

**Mental Health Consumer
Advocacy Organizations**
Anxiety Disorders Association
  of America
Dept. B
P.O. Box 96505
Washington, DC 20077-7140
(301) 231-9350

Freedom From Fear
308 Seaview Avenue
Staten Island, NY 10305
(718) 351-1717

National Anxiety Foundation
3135 Custer Drive
Lexington, KY 40517
(606) 272-7166

National Alliance for the Mentally Ill
2101 Wilson Boulevard, Suite 302
Arlington, VA 22201
(800) 950-6264

National Institute of Mental Health
Information Resources and Inquiries Branch/Publication List
Room 15C-05
5600 Fishers Lane
Rockville, MD 20857
(301) 443-4513

National Mental Health Association
1201 Prince Street
Alexandria, VA 22314-2971
(703) 684-7722

National Panic/Anxiety Disorder Newsletter
1718 Burgundy Place, Suite B
Santa Rosa, CA 95403
(707) 527-5738

Selective Mutism Foundation
c/o Sue Leszcyk
P.O. Box 450632
Sunrise, FL 33345-0632
(305) 748-7714 (tel/fax)

Centers for Social Phobia Research

The following universities and hospitals are some of the centers of ongoing research into social anxiety and social phobia. These centers may offer treatment studies for eligible persons, and they may also make referrals to local experts.

California

University of California, San Diego
Psychopharmacology Research Program
8950 Villa La Jolla Drive #2243
La Jolla, CA 92037
(619) 622-6111

Palo Alto Shyness Clinic
407 Burgess Drive
Menlo Park, CA 94025
(415) 328-6115

Iowa

Anxiety Clinic
Department of Psychiatry
University of Iowa Hospital and Clinics
200 Hawkins Drive
Iowa City, IA 52242
(319) 353-6314

Massachusetts

Anxiety Clinic and Research Program at Massachusetts General Hospital
15 Parkman Street #815
Boston, MA 02114
(617) 726-3488

Michigan
Anxiety Disorders Program
University of Michigan, Department of Psychiatry
1500 East Medical Center Drive
Ann Arbor, MI 48109-0840
(313) 764-5348

Department of Psychiatry
Wayne State University Health Center
4201 St. Antoine 9B
Detroit, MI 48201
(313) 577-6463

Missouri
Anxiety Disorders Center
St. Louis University Medical Sciences Center
1221 South Grand Boulevard
St. Louis, MO 63104
(314) 577-8718

Nebraska
Psychological Consultation Center
111 Burnett Hall
University of Nebraska
Lincoln, NE 68588-0311
(402) 472-2351

New York
Anxiety Disorders Clinic (at Columbia-Presbyterian Medical Center)
New York State Psychiatric Institute
722 West 168th Street
New York, NY 10032
(212) 960-2367

Social Phobia Program
Center for Stress and Anxiety Disorders
State University of New York
1535 Western Avenue
Albany, NY 12203
(518) 442-4822

North Carolina
Anxiety and Traumatic Stress Program
Duke University Medical Center
Box 3812
Durham, NC 27710
(919) 684-2880

Pennsylvania
Center for the Treatment and Study of Anxiety
Medical College of Pennsylvania
Department of Psychiatry
3200 Henry Avenue
Philadelphia, PA 19129
(215) 842-4010

Department of Psychology
Temple University
Weiss Hall
Philadelphia, PA 19140
(215) 204-1575

Anxiety Disorders Program
Western Psychiatric Institute and Clinic
3811 O'Hara Street
Pittsburgh, PA 15213
(412) 624-5500

South Carolina
Anxiety Prevention, Treatment
and Research Center
Institute of Psychiatry at the
Medical University of South
Carolina
171 Ashley Avenue
Charleston, SC 29425
(803) 792-5900
(803) 792-4100

Texas
Laboratory for the Study of Anx-
iety Disorders
Department of Psychology
University of Texas
Austin, TX 78712
(512) 471-5177

Wisconsin
Dean Foundation for Health, Education and Research
8000 Excelsior Drive
Suite 302
Madison, WI 52717
(608) 836-8030

Canada
Anxiety Disorders Clinic
Chedoke-McMaster Hospital
McMaster Division
1200 Main Street West
Hamilton, Ontario L8N 3Z5
(905) 521-5018

St. Mary's Hospital
Montreal, Quebec H3T 1M5
(514) 345-3584

Royal University Hospital
Anxiety and Mood Disorders
Program
Department of Psychiatry, Room
#111 Ellis Hall
Saskatoon, Saskatchewan S7N
0X0
(306) 966-8226

The Clarke Institute of
Psychiatry
250 College Street
Toronto, Ontario M5T 1R 8
(416) 979-2221

Anxiety Disorders Clinic
St. Boniface Hospital
Winnipeg, Manitoba R2H 2A6
(204) 237-2606

**Nonprofessional Program for
Public Speaking Skills**
Toastmasters International
P.O. Box 10400
Santa Ana, CA 92711
(714) 542-6793

**Social Anxiety Information on
the Internet**
Alt.support.social-phobia
(news and support)

http://www.albany.edu/pr/
anxiety1.html
(State University of New York
at Albany home page:
includes information on social
phobia research)

http://www.chesulwind.com/
    parents
(Parenting Solutions: help for
    childhood problems, including
    shyness)

http://www.chesulwind.com/
    shyness
(Information on shyness from
    Drs. Schneier and Welkowitz)

http://www.shyness.com/
(The Palo Alto Shyness Clinic:
    information on research and
    private consultations)

BIBLIOGRAPHY

Chapter 1

Kessler, R. C.; McGonagle, K. A.; Zhao, S.; Nelson, C. B.; Hughes, M.; Eshelman, S.; Wittchen, H.; and Kendler, K. S. (1994). Lifetime and 12-month prevalence of DSM-III-R psychiatric disorders in the United States. *Archives of General Psychiatry, 51,* 8–19.

Liebowitz, M. R.; Gorman, J. M.; Fyer, A. J.; and Klein, D. F. (1985). Social phobia: Review of a neglected anxiety disorder. *Archives of General Psychiatry, 42,* 729–736.

Chapter 2

American Psychiatric Association. (1994). *Diagnostic and Statistical Manual of Mental Disorders (DSM-IV), 4th ed.* Washington, D.C.: American Psychiatric Association.

Burton, R. (1621). *The Anatomy of Melancholy (11th ed. 1813, vol. 1),* (p. 272). London.

Caspi, A.; Elder, G. H., Jr.; and Bem, D. J. (1988). Moving away from the world: Life-course patterns of shy children. *Developmental Psychology, 24,* 824–831.

Janet, P. (1903). *Les obsessions et la psychastenie.* Paris: Alcan.

Kessler, R. C.; McGonagle, K. A.; Zhao, S.; Nelson, C. B.; Hughes, M.; Eshelman, S.; Wittchen, H.; and Kendler, K. S. (1994). Lifetime and 12-month prevalence of DSM-III-R psychiatric disorders in the United States. *Archives of General Psychiatry, 51,* 8–19.

Marks, I. (1970). The classification of phobic disorders. *British Journal of Psychiatry, 116,* 377–386.

Schneier, F. R.; Johnson, J.; Hornig, C. D.; Liebowitz, M. R.; and Weissman, M. M. (1992). Social phobia: Comorbidity and morbid-

ity in an epidemiological sample. *Archives of General Psychiatry,
49,* 282–288.

Stein, M. B.; Walker, J. R.; and Forde, D. R. (1994). Setting diagnostic
thresholds for social phobia: Considerations from a community survey of social anxiety. *American Journal of Psychiatry, 151,*
408–412.

Turner, S. M.; Beidel, D. C.; Dancu, C. V.; and Keys, D. J. (1986).
Psychopathology of social phobia and comparison to avoidant personality disorder. *Journal of Abnormal Psychology, 95,* 389–394.

Chapter 6
Darwin, Charles. (1873). *The Expression of Emotion in Man and Ani-
mals,* (pp. 312–314). London: Murray. (Reprinted 1965. Chicago:
University of Chicago Press.)

Chapter 8
Abramovitch, R. (1976). The relationship of attention and proximity
to rank in preschool children. In M. R. Chance and R. R. Larsen,
eds. *The Social Structure of Attention,* (pp. 153–176). London: John
Wiley and Sons.

Cook, M., and Mineka, S. (1991). Selective associations in the origins
of phobic fears and their implications for behavior therapy. In P.
Martin, ed. *Handbook of Behavior Therapy and Psychological Science: An Integrative Approach,* (pp. 413–434). Elmsford, N.Y.: Per-
gamon Press.

Darwin, Charles. (1873). *The Expression of Emotion in Man and Animals* (p. 309). London: Murray. (Reprinted 1965. Chicago: University of Chicago Press.)

DeWaal, F. B. M. (1982). *Chimpanzee Politics: Power and Sex Among
the Apes,* (pp. 49–50, 133). New York: Harper and Row.

Diderot, Denis. (1796). *Supplement au Voyage de Bougainville.* (Reprinted 1972. New York: French and European Publications.)

Gilbert, P. (1989). *Human Nature and Suffering.* Hove, Sussex: Lawrence Erlbaum Associates.

Goodall, Jane. (1986). *The Chimpanzees of Gombe,* (pp. 184, 325, 361,
437). Cambridge, Mass.: Belknap Press of Harvard University Press.

Leary, M. R.; Britt, T. W.; Cutlip, W. D.; and Templeton, J. L. (1992).
Social blushing. *Psychological Bulletin, 112,* 446–460.

Miller, Jean Baker. (1986). *Toward a New Psychology of Women.* 4th
ed., (pp. 38–43). Boston: Beacon Press.

Öhman, A. (1986). Face the beast and fear the face: Animal and social fears as prototypes for evolutionary analyses of emotion. *Psychophysiology, 23,* 123–145.

Schlenker, B., and Leary, M. (1985). Social anxiety and communication about the self. *Journal of Language & Social Psychology, 4,* 171–192.

Scott, J. P. (1977). Agonistic behavior. In M. T. McGuire and L. A. Fairbanks, eds. *Ethological Psychiatry,* (pp. 193–210). New York: Grune and Stratton.

Seligman, M. E. P., and Hager, J. L. (1971). *Biological Boundaries of Learning.* Englewood Cliffs, N.J.: Prentice-Hall.

Tannen, Deborah. (1990). *You Just Don't Understand,* (pp. 62–63). New York: Ballantine Books.

Chapter 9

Biederman, J.; Rosenbaum, J. F.; Bolduc-Murphy, E. A.; Faraone, S. V.; Challoff, J.; Hirshfeld, D. R.; and Kagan, J. (1993). A 3-year follow-up of children with and without behavioral inhibition. *Journal of the American Academy of Child and Adolescent Psychiatry, 32,* 814–821.

Bremner, J. D.; Randall, P.; Scott, T. M.; Bronen, R. A.; Seibyl, J. P.; Southwick, S. M.; Delaney, R. C.; McCarthy, G.; Charney, D. S.; and Innis, R. B. (1995). MRI-based measurement of hippocampal volume in patients with combat-related posttraumatic stress disorder. *American Journal of Psychiatry, 152,* 973–981.

Fyer, A. J.; Mannuzza, S.; Chapman, T. F.; Martin, L.Y.; and Klein, D. F. (1995). Specificity in familial aggregation of phobic disorders. *Archives of General Psychiatry, 52,* 564–573.

Higley, J. D.; Suomi, S. J.; and Linnoila, M. (1990). Developmental influences on the serotonergic system and timidity in the nonhuman primate. In E. F. Coccaro and D. L. Murphy, eds. *Developmental Influences on the Serotonergic System and Timidity in the Nonhuman Primate,* (pp. 29–46). Washington, D.C.: American Psychiatric Press, Inc.

James, William. (1950). *Principles of Psychology.* New York: Dover. Originally published 1890.

Kagan, J. (1989). Temperamental contributions to social behavior. *American Psychologist, 44,* 668–674.

———. (1994). *Galen's Prophecy,* (pp. 122–135, 173–193). New York: Basic Books.

Keltner, D. (1995). Signs of appeasement: Evidence for the distinct displays of embarrassment, amusement, and shame. *Journal of Personality and Social Psychology, 3,* 441–454.

Kendler, K. S.; Neale, M. C.; Kessler, R. C.; Heath, A. C.; and Eaves, L. J. (1992). The genetic epidemiology of phobias in women: The interrelations of agoraphobia, social phobia, situational phobia and simple phobia. *Archives of General Psychiatry, 49,* 273–281.

Levin, A. P.; Saoud, J. B.; Strauman, T.; Gorman, J. M.; Fyer, A. J.; Crawford, R.; and Liebowitz, M. R. (1993). Responses of "generalized" and "discrete" social phobics during public speaking. *Journal of Anxiety Disorders, 7,* 207–221.

Liebowitz, M. R.; Campeas, R.; and Hollander, E. (1987). Possible dopamine dysregulation in social phobia and atypical depression, (letter). *Psychiatry Research, 22,* 89–90.

Mayleben, M. A.; Gariepy, J.-L.; Tancer, M. E.; et al. (1992). Genetic differences in social behavior: Neurobiological mechanisms in a mouse model, (abstract). *Biological Psychiatry, 31,* 216A.

Papp, L. A.; Gorman, J. M.; Liebowitz, M. R.; Fyer, A. J.; Cohen, B.; and Klein, D. F. (1988). Epinephrine infusions in patients with social phobia. *American Journal of Psychiatry, 145,* 733–736.

Potts, N. L. S.; Davidson, J. R. T.; and Krishnan, K. R. R. (1994). Magnetic resonance imaging in social phobia. *Psychiatry Research, 52,* 35–42.

Raleigh, M. J.; McGuire, M. T.; Brammer, G. L.; Pollack, D. B.; and Yuwiler, A. (1991). Serotonergic mechanisms promote dominance acquisition in adult male vervet monkeys. *Brain Research, 559,* 181–190.

Rosenbaum, J. F.; Biederman, J.; Hirshfeld, D. R.; Bolduc, E. A.; Faraone, S. V.; Kagan, J.; Snidman, N.; and Reznik, J. S. (1991). Further evidence of an association between behavioral inhibition and anxiety disorders: Results from a family study of children from a non-clinical sample. *Journal of Psychiatry Research, 25,* 49–65.

Schachter, S., and Singer, J. E. (1962). Cognitive, social and physiological determinants of emotional state. *Psychology Review, 69,* 370–399.

Stein, M. R.; Heuser, I. J.; Juncos, J. L.; and Uhde, T. W. (1990). Anxiety disorders in patients with Parkinson's disease. *American Journal of Psychiatry, 147,* 207–210.

Yehuda, R.; Kahana, B.; Binder-Brynes, K.; Southwick, S. M.; Mason, J. W.; and Giller, E. L. (1995). Low urinary cortisol excretion in Holocaust survivors with posttraumatic stress disorder. *American Journal of Psychiatry, 152,* 982–986.

Chapter 10

Allamen, J.; Joyce, C.; and Crandell, V. (1972). The antecedents of social desirability response tendencies of children and young adults. *Child Development, 43,* 1135–1160.

Bowlby, J. (1969). *Attachment.* London: Hogarth Press.

Breuer, J., and Freud, S. (1955). Studies on hysteria. In J. Strachey, ed. and trans. *The Standard Edition of the Complete Psychological Works of Sigmund Freud, (vol. 2, pp. vii–xxxi, 1–311).* London: Hogarth Press. (Original work published 1893–1895.)

Ellis, A. (1962). *Reason and Emotion in Psychotherapy.* New York: Lyle Stuart.

Engfer, A. (1993). Antecedents and consequences of shyness in boys and girls: A 6-year longitudinal study. In K. H. Rubin and J. B. Asendorpf, eds. *Social Withdrawal, Inhibition, and Shyness in Childhood,* (pp. 49–79). Hillsdale, N.J.: Erlbaum.

Gabbard, Glen O. (1983). Further contributions to the understanding of stage fright: Narcissistic issues. *Journal of the American Psychoanalytic Association, 31,* 423–431.

Jung, C. G. (1954–1971). Psychological typology. In G. Adler, ed., R. F. Hull, trans. *The Collected Works of C. G. Jung,* (vol. 6, pp. 550–551). Princeton: Princeton University Press. (Original work published 1936.)

Lang, P. (1993). The three-system approach to emotion. In N. Birbaumer and A. Öhman, eds. *The Structure of Emotion,* (pp. 18–30). Seattle, Wash.: Hogrefe and Huber.

Mineka, S., and Zinbarg, R. (1995). In R. G. Heimberg, M. R. Liebowitz, D. A. Hope, and F. R. Schneier, eds. *Social Phobia: Diagnosis, Assessment, and Treatment,* (pp. 134–162).

Ost, L., and Hugdahl, K. (1981). Acquisition of phobias and anxiety response patterns in clinical patients. *Behaviour Research and Therapy, 16,* 439–447.

Parker, G. (1979). Reported parental characteristics of agoraphobics and social phobics. *British Journal of Psychiatry, 135,* 555–560.

Schlenker, B., and Leary, M. (1982). Social anxiety and self-presentation: A conceptualization and model. *Psychological Bulletin, 92,* 641–669.

Skinner, B. F. (1953). *Science and Human Behavior.* New York: Free Press.

Stopa, Luisa, and Clark, David. (1993). Cognitive processes in social phobia. *Behavior Research and Therapy, 31,* no. 3, 255–267.

Watson, J. B. and Rayner, R. (1920). Conditioned emotional reactions. *Journal of Experimental Psychology, 3,* 319–324.

Chapter 11

Bateson, M. C. (1989). *Composing a Life.* New York: Atlantic Monthly Press.

Chaleby, Kutaiba. (1987). Social phobia in Saudis. *Social Psychiatry, 22,* 167–170.

Darwin, Charles. (1873). *The Expression of Emotion in Man and Animals,* (pp. 315–320). London: Murray. (Reprinted 1965. Chicago: University of Chicago Press.)

Edelmann, Robert J.; Asendorpf, J.; Contarello, A.; Zammuner, V.; Georgas, J.; and Villanueva, C. (1989). Self-reported expression of embarrassment in five European cultures. *Journal of Cross-Cultural Psychology, 20* (4), 357–371.

Funicello, Annette, and Romanowski, Patricia. (1994). *A Dream Is a Wish Your Heart Makes: My Story,* (p. 114). New York: Hyperion.

Goffman, Erving. (1959). *The Presentation of Self in Everyday Life.* Garden City, N.Y.: Doubleday Anchor Books, Doubleday and Co., Inc.

Guida, F. V., and Ludlow, L. H. (1989). A cross-cultural study of test anxiety. *Journal of Cross-Cultural Psychology, 20, (2),* 178–190.

Schneier, F. R.; Johnson, J.; Hornig, C. D.; Liebowitz, M. R.; and Weissman, M. M. (1992). Social phobia: Comorbidity and morbidity in an epidemiological sample. *Archives of General Psychiatry, 49,* 282–288.

Shweder, R. A. (1993). The cultural psychology of the emotions. In M. Lewis and J. M. Haviland, eds. *Handbook of Emotions,* (pp. 417–431). New York: Guilford Press.

Takahashi, Tooru. (1989). Social phobia syndrome in Japan. *Comprehensive Psychiatry, 30,* 45–52.

Chapter 12

Adams, C. (1986). Misha the magnificent: A very intimate interview with ballet's brightest (and sexiest) star. *Ladies' Home Journal,* December, 20–24, 162.

Barich, B. (1993). Still truckin'. *The New Yorker,* October 11, 96–102.

Clark, D. B., and Agras, W. S. (1991). The assessment and treatment of performance anxiety in musicians. *American Journal of Psychiatry, 148,* 598–605.

Corredor, J. M. (1956). *Conversations with Casals.* New York: Dutton.

Feldman, L. (1991). Strikeouts and psych-outs. *New York Times Magazine,* July 7, 10–13, 30.

Leo, J. (1983). Take me out to the ballgame. *Time,* August 15, 72.

Olivier, Laurence. (1982). *Confessions of an Actor,* (pp. 217–218). London: George Weidenfeld and Nicholson Limited.

Price, S. (1994). Barbra's fight against fear. *Ladies' Home Journal,* July, 109–111, 156–160.

Seligman, J.; Namuth, T.; and Miller, M. (1994). Drowning on dry land. *Newsweek,* May 23, 64–66.

Thayer, L. (1995). Applause, applause: Anyone can win over a tough audience. Just ask Lee Iacocca. *Effective Focus,* October, 17–18.

Vanity Fair. (1994). Streisand. November, 153–159, 190–194.

Wilson, Glenn D. (1994). *Psychology for Performing Artists: Butterflies and Bouquets.* London: Jessica Kingsley Publishers Ltd.

Chapter 13

Barlow, D. H. (1986). Causes of sexual dysfunction: The role of anxiety and cognitive interference. *Journal of Consulting and Clinical Psychology, 54,* 140–148.

Darwin, Charles. (1873). *The Expression of Emotion in Man and Animals,* (p. 336). London: Murray. (Reprinted 1965. Chicago: University of Chicago Press.)

Hunter, John. (1786). A treatise on the venereal disease, London [for the author], pp. 200–204. In R. Hunter and I. Macalpine, eds., (pp. 493–494). *Three Hundred Years of Psychiatry 1535–1860.* (1982). Hartsdale, N.Y.: Carlisle Publishing Inc.

Leary, M. R., and Dobbins, S. E. (1983). Social anxiety, sexual behavior, and contraceptive use. *Journal of Personality and Social Psychiatry, 43,* 1347–1354.

Masters, W. H., and Johnson, V. E. (1970). *Human Sexual Inadequacy.* London: Little, Brown and Co.

Yeazell, R. B. (1984). *Fictions of Modesty,* (p. 74). Chicago: University of Chicago Press.

Zimbardo, P. G. (1977). *Shyness: What It Is, What to Do About It,* (pp. 94–95). New York: Addison-Wesley.

Chapter 14

La Greca, A.; Dandes, S.; Wick, P.; Shaw, K.; and Stone, W. (1988). Development of the Social Anxiety Scale for Children: Reliability and concurrent validity. *Journal of Clinical and Child Psychology, 17,* 84–91.

Leary, M. (1983). Social anxiousness: The construct and its measurement. *Journal of Personality Assessment, 47,* 66–75.

Liebowitz, M. R. (1987). Social Phobia. *Modern Problems of Pharmacopsychiatry, 22,* 141–173.

Paul, G. (1966). *Insight vs Desensitization in Psychotherapy.* Stanford, Calif.: Stanford University Press.

Schneier, F.; Heckelman, L.; Garfinkel, R.; Campeas, R.; Fallon, B.; Gitow, A.; Street, L.; Del Bene, D.; and Liebowitz, M. (1994). Functional impairment in Social Phobia. *Journal of Clinical Psychiatry, 55*(8), 322–331.

Chapter 17

Baumrind, D. (1980). New directions in socialization research. *American Psychologist, 35,* 639–652.

Black, B., and Uhde, T. W. (1995). Psychiatric characteristics of children with selective mutism: A pilot study. *Journal of the American Academy of Child and Adolescent Psychiatry, 34 (7),* 847–856.

Boon, F. (1994). The selective mutism controversy. *Journal of the American Academy of Child and Adolescent Psychiatry, 33,* 283.

Caspi, A.; Elder, G. H., Jr.; and Bem, D. J. (1988). Moving away from the world: Life-course patterns of shy children. *Developmental Psychology, 24,* 824–831.

Dow, S.; Sonies, B.; Scheib, D.; Moss, S.; and Leonard, H. (1995). Practical guidelines for the assessment and treatment of selective mutism. *Journal of the American Academy of Child and Adolescent Psychiatry, 34* (7), 836–846.

Griffin, S. (1995). A cognitive-developmental analysis of pride, shame, and embarrassment in middle childhood. In J. P. Tangney and K. W. Fischer, eds. *Self-conscious Emotions,* (pp. 219–236). New York: Guilford Press.

Johnson, R. L., and Glass, C. R. (1989). Heterosocial anxiety and direction of attention in high school boys. *Cognitive Therapy and Research, 13,* 509–526.

Kagan, J.; Snidman, N.; and Arcus, D. (1993). On the temperamental categories of inhibited and uninhibited children. In K. H. Rubin and J. B. Asendorpf, eds. *Social Withdrawal, Inhibition, and Shyness in Childhood,* (pp. 19–28). Hillsdale, N.J.: Erlbaum.

Kandel, D. B.; Kessler, R. C.; and Margulies, R. Z. (1978). Antecedents of adolescent initiation into stages of drug use: A developmental analysis. *Journal of Youth and Adolescence, 7,* 13–40.

Rubin, K. H.; LeMare, L.; and Lollis, S. (1990). Social withdrawal in childhood: Developmental pathways to rejection. In S. R. Asher and J. D. Coie, eds. *Peer Rejection in Childhood,* (pp. 217–249). New York: Cambridge University Press.

Strauss, C. C.; Frame, C. L.; and Forehand, R. (1987). Psychosocial impairment associated with anxiety in children. *Journal of Clinical Child Psychology, 16,* 235–239.

Thomas, A.; Chess, S.; and Birch, H. G. (1970). The origin of personality. *Scientific American, 223,* 102–109.

Chapter 18

Consumer Reports. (1995). Mental health: Does therapy help? November, 734–739.

Heimberg, R. G.; Dodge, C. S.; Hope, D. A.; Kennedy, C. R.; Zollo, L. J.; and Becker, R. E. (1990). Cognitive behavioral treatment for social phobia: Comparison with credible placebo control. *Cognitive Therapy and Research, 14,* 1–23.

Heimberg, R. G.; Salzman, D. G.; Holt, C. S.; and Blendel, K. A. (1993). Cognitive behavioral group treatment for social phobia: Effectiveness at five-year follow-up. *Cognitive Therapy and Research, 17,* 325–339.

Moreno, J. (1969). *Psychodrama. Vol. 3, Action Therapy and Principle of Practice.* New York: Beacon House.

Sossin, K., and Loman, S. (1992). Clinical applications of the Kestenberg Movement Profile. In S. Loman, ed., *The Body-Mind Connection in Human Movement Analysis.* Keene, N.H.: Antioch New England.

Turner, S. M.; Beidel, D. C.; Cooley, M. R.; Woody, S. R.; and Messer, S. C. (1994). A multicomponent behavioral treatment for social phobia: Social Effectiveness Therapy. *Behaviour Research and Therapy, 32,* 381–390.

Turner, S. M.; Beidel, D. C.; and Jacob, R. G. (1994). Social phobia: A comparison of behavior therapy and atenolol. *Journal of Consulting and Clinical Psychology, 62,* 350–358.

Wilson, Glenn D. (1994). *Psychology for Performing Artists: Butterflies and Bouquets.* London: Jessica Kingsley Publishers Ltd.

Chapter 19

Baxter, L. R., Jr.; Schwartz, J. M.; Bergman, K. S.; Szuba, M. P.; Guze, B. H.; Mazziotta, J. C.; Alazraki, A.; Selin, C. E.; Ferng, H.-K.; Munford, P.; and Phelps, M. E. (1992). Caudate glucose metabolic rate changes with both drug and behavioral therapy for obsessive-compulsive disorder. *Archives of General Psychiatry, 49,* 681–689.

Black, B., and Uhde, T. W. (1994). Treatment of elective mutism with fluoxetine: a double-blind, placebo-controlled study. *Journal of the*

American Academy of Child and Adolescent Psychiatry, 33, 1000–1006.

Davidson, J. R. T.; Potts, N. L. S.; Richichi, E.; Krishnan, K. R. R.; Ford, S. M.; Smith, R.; and Wilson, W. H. (1993). Treatment of social phobia with clonazepam and placebo. *Journal of Clinical Psychopharmacology, 13,* 423–429.

Fishbein, M.; Middlestadt, S. E.; Ottati, V.; Straus, S.; and Ellis, A. (1988). Medical problems among ICSOM. *Problems of Performing Artists, 3,* 1–8.

Kramer, Peter D. (1993). *Listening to Prozac,* (pp. 7–11). New York: Viking.

Liebowitz, M. R.; Gorman, J. M.; Fyer, A. J.; and Klein, D. F. (1985). Social phobia: Review of a neglected anxiety disorder. *Archives of General Psychiatry, 42,* 729–736.

Schneier, F. R. (1995). Monoamine oxidase inhibitors, selective serotonin reuptake inhibitors, and other antidepressants in pharmacotherapy. In Stein, M. R., ed. *Social Phobia: Clinical and Research Perspectives* (pp. 347–374). Washington, D.C.: American Psychiatric Association Press.

Schneier, F. R.; Marshall, R. D.; Street, L.; and Heimberg, R. (1995). Social phobia and specific phobias. In Gabbard, G. O., ed. *Treatments of Psychiatric Disorders.* Vol. 2. 2nd ed. (pp. 1453–1476). Washington, D.C.: American Psychiatric Association Press.

Chapter 20

Gates, Bill. (1995). *The Road Ahead.* New York: Viking, (p. 206).

Jones, S. G. (1995). *Cybersociety: Computer Mediated Communication and Community.* Thousand Oaks, Calif.: Sage.

INDEX

A

Adolescents, 199–201
  alcohol and, 204
  cognitive-behavioral self-help
    approach for, 200
  drugs and, 204
  meta-conversations with, 201–3
  when to seek professional
    help for, 204
Adrenaline:
  hypothesis concerning, 72–73
  normal role of, 219
Agoraphobia, 231
Alcoholism, 17, 18, 30
  adolescents and, 204
Alexander technique, 213
Alprazolam, 223
Amygdala, 62
Anafranil (clomipramine), 235
Animal behavior:
  level of self-consciousness, 53
  social ranking, 51–52
  submission, 52–53
Animals, fear of, 48–50
Anxiety. *See* Social anxiety
Anxiety Disorders Association
  of America, 214, 243

Aristotle, 81
Asia, Southern, social fears in,
  106
Assertive option, 168–69
Authority figures, dealing with, 15
Avoidant personality disorder, 19

B

Barlow, David, sexual perfor-
    mance anxiety studies, 128
Baryshnikov, Mikhail, 120
Bateson, Mary Catherine, 111
Behavorial inhibition, 68–71
  early identification of, 68–71
Behavorial psychology, 82–83
Beidel, Deborah, 208, 209
Benzodiazepines, 75, 222–23,
    235
  controversy concerning, 225
  effectiveness, 223–24
  how they work, 223
  limitations, 224
  side effects, 224
Beta-blockers, 73, 121–22, 218,
    235

H

Heart rate reactions, 74
Heights, fear of, 49
Heimberg, Richard, 148, 208
Hippocrates, 13
Human behavior:
  competition and cooperation,
    54–56
  environmental factors concern-
    ing, 58
  evolution factors concerning,
    57–58
  submission, 56–57
Hunter, John, early therapy for
  sexual performance anxiety,
  129–30
Hysteroid dysphoric, 230–31

I

Immigrants, 107–9
Inderal (propranolol), 218
Inhibited temperament, 68–71
Insight-oriented therapy, 211–12
Interacting, fears of, self-test for,
  136–37
Interaction Anxiousness Scale,
  136–37
Introversion, 97–98

J

Jackson, Glenda, 119–20
James, William, 71–72
James-Lange theory, 71–72
Janet, Pierre, 13
Japan, social fears in, 103–5
Jones, Steve, 246

Jung, C. G., on personality
  types, 97–98

K

Kagan, Jerome, inhibited temper-
  ament study, 68–71
Keats, John, 36
Kendler, Kenneth, twins study,
  67–68
Klein, Donald, 230
Klonopin (clonazepam), 75, 223
Kramer, Peter, 228

L

Lang, Peter, three-system model,
  92–93
Lange, Carl, 71–72
Layja, 106
Leary, Mark, 56, 88
  Interaction Anxiousness Scale,
    136–37
Liebowitz, Michael, 231
  hypothesis concerning dopa-
    mine, 75–77
Liebowitz Disability Self-Rating
  Scale, 140–42
Liebowitz Social Anxiety Scale,
  138–40
Life experiences, 65
  biological tendencies and,
    64–65
  negative, 65
Listening to Prozac (Kramer),
  228
Luvox (fluvoxamine), 226

T

ABOUT THE AUTHORS

FRANKLIN SCHNEIER, M.D. is associate director of the Anxiety Disorders Clinic at New York State Psychiatric Institute and associate professor of clinical psychiatry at the College of Physicians and Surgeons of Columbia University. He is author of more than 40 articles on social phobia and other anxiety disorders, and he is an editor of the book *Social Phobia: Diagnosis, Assessment, and Treatment.* Dr. Schneier lectures on anxiety disorders and maintains a private practice in New York City.

LAWRENCE WELKOWITZ, Ph.D. is a research psychologist at the New York State Psychiatric Institute and Columbia University. He has published numerous papers on behavioral therapies for difficult problems including phobias, anxiety, and self-destructive behavior. He has private practices in New York City and Keene, New Hampshire.